Acknowledgements

I was able to write this with the help of partners at Ochsner Clinic Foundation. Dr. Carl Lavie and his colleagues shared cutting edge knowledge in cardiology. Drs. Lillian Lesser and Morris Burka helped me edit the mental health section. I also paraphrased what I learned at a Harvard Review course, Understanding Men and Boys. Dr. John Phipps helped me write the alcoholism chapter. Dr. Howard Woo helped with the urology section, Dr. Troy Scroggins with the prostate cancer parts, Dr. Jill Lindberg with the kidney stone portion, and Dr. Al Burshell of Endocrinology helped me with the diabetes and testosterone sections. Dr. Franz Messerli of Hypertension at Ochsner helped me with the hypertension chapter.

A special thanks to Dr. Mike Wilson for his wonderful stories and wit. He helped me make this humorous even though it is all true.

We will always hold the doctors at Mayo Clinic who taught us the art and science of medicine, in highest esteem. As Mayo Clinic trained doctors, we were positioned to help many patients through the years. Our training was second to none.

I thank Joy Parker for editing the first version, and Dr. Don Rugg and Dr. and Mrs. J.M. Woodhouse for reading it and giving me feedback. I thank Chris Wiltz for her ideas on how to present the material. Thanks to Rebecca O'Meara for her creative business promotion and marketing ideas and to Stephanie Robison of Upside Design for her witty cover design.

A special thanks to Robert L. Bach in Minneapolis, the attorney who has watched over this project and kept us out of trouble.

Disclaimer

Everything I wrote I currently believe to be true and this is how I practice medicine for midlife men. But in medicine, we are always questioning what we believe, so some of the information could become outdated. (I'll need to write an updated version in the future.)

Although this information is generally helpful, I am not prescribing what any individual should do. He must consult with his own doctor because everyone's situation is different. The contents of the book are my professional opinion and I do not pretend to speak for other doctors. I do not intend this book as a standard of care reference.

The persons in the stories are disguised so there is no way that anyone can recognize himself, except for the few instances where a generous patient has said to me, "If I can help someone else with my story, please tell it."

YOUR HUSBAND'S HEALTH:
Simplify Your Worry List

TABLE OF CONTENTS

INTRODUCTION

I Wrote This Book to Let You Cross Some Things Off Your Worry List

I am a wife like you. I have been married thirty years. More than ever, my life and future intertwines with my husband as we try to finish out our careers and plan for retirement. I watch over his health and well-being like a hawk. It occurred to me that you would do the same for your husband and that you probably want the same facts that I have.

I am writing this book to empower you, not to frighten you about all the unknowable scary things like SARS and mad cow disease and West Nile virus. Most men aren't stricken by these media popular conditions. Most men are laid low by heart attacks, stroke, or cancer.

Then there are those nagging worries. As our husbands put on a little age, or their hair thins, they worry about themselves or get depressed, but can't acknowledge any weakness, no matter how much it gnaws at them, without appearing unmanly. So what do you do for your husband if he gained twenty pounds, seems depressed, or can't get an erection?

In the last three years, our generation saw the fall in the stock market, the drop in the value of our retirement plans, the prospect of unemployment and competition from younger, less expensive workers, and the unstable world situation including another war with Iraq. While there is little we can do about those things, there is a lot we can do to help each other be healthier; and to live better lives. We may have little control over the cost of medical insurance, but we can control our own health costs to a large extent by understanding how disease happens and what we can do to prevent illness and catastrophes.

The other reason I needed to write this book for you is the difficulty of the current medical system. I am not going to pretend to you that it functions well. Many doctors don't have the knowledge I will impart to you in this book because the system is focused on the many very ill people. And yet midlife people are at an age when they can often avoid the illnesses plaguing older adults. Most people our age get a short time with a doctor every other year and in that time, the doctor can't do a physical, complete the paperwork for tests, fill out insurance forms, and explain what you really need to know about your present condition and how to prevent future health problems. Even if your doctor is well meaning, the system forces him or her to see more and more patients in the same amount of time with less help.

You need to have the information in this book to protect your husband, your marriage, your family and your assets. You can no longer be certain that your doctor is able to watch over you personally, keep up on the medical knowledge that impacts your age group, or that you will even have the same doctor from year to year if your workplace changes HMOs.

The Nightmare

The woman is already stressed to the max. She has a full time job, children including a teenager who is acting out, and aging parents who need her time as they are less able to care for themselves. She and her husband have a monthly mortgage and a college tuition payment and haven't been able to save much. Their company's pension plan just changed to defined contribution so their retirement savings are nowhere near what they need. They have both reached the top of their earning potential, but in the last few years, several of their co-workers were given the pink slip, so now they do the work of two people for the same salary. She doesn't get enough sleep, exercise, or any peace and quiet.

One day she comes home to an empty kitchen; his coat is hanging there; his smell is still on the pillow in the bed; his dirty shorts are in a pile in the bathroom waiting for her to pick them up. She has this sinking feeling that he may have walked out on their stressful life together. Then she goes into the den and at first she thinks she sees him lying asleep in his Lazy Boy chair, while a ball game blares in the background. She tries to rouse him from the sleep, panicking when she realizes he's not breathing; frantically calling 911; trying to wake him up, trying to remember CPR. She had tried to get him to go to the doctor but he kept putting it off, saying he felt fine.

I am going to tell you how these things happen and what you can do so they do not happen to your husband in the middle of your lives together.

Who I Am

Since 1993 I have been an internal (adult) medicine doctor at the internationally respected Ochsner Clinic Foundation in New Orleans. Ochsner Clinic Foundation is a group practice of over four hundred staff physicians and two hundred and fifty resident physicians in training. We have doctors in all specialties and subspecialties practicing in one large clinic, and thirty smaller neighborhood clinics, with over a million patient visits annually, a six hundred-bed hospital, operating rooms, an emergency room, critical care units, laboratories and radiology.

As an internist, I see close to five thousand patients a year, ages eighteen to one hundred. My patients come from all walks of life, and are as racially diverse as this magical port city of New Orleans. African-Americans, Vietnamese, Hispanics, Caucasians of all ethnic mixtures, Cajuns (French-Canadians who moved to Louisiana over one hundred years ago), New Orleanians from old families, Yankees (a lot of us live and work in New Orleans and love our city), and Islamic and Hindu patients are all under my care.

I write about what I have learned from Mayo Clinic training, my patients, colleagues, medical journals, and Harvard review courses. Ongoing study is crucial to competent medical practice. By its very nature, science is always questioning if what we think we know is really true. The flip flops are frustrating to the public but necessary to the scientific process by which we ferret out the facts.

I entered medical school in 1971 at the University of Iowa. In medical school, we learned how to take care of patients and got a handle on what we would need to know to be good doctors. In 1975 I went to Mayo Clinic for my three year internal medicine residency and two year gastroenterology fellowship. I cannot imagine any better medical training than what I received from the doctors at Mayo Clinic. There was little else to do during those long Minnesota winters except see patients and study in the magnificent Mayo library.

From 1985 to 1993, I was on active duty in the Air Force as Chief of Executive Medicine and doctor to the General Officers and their wives, those on active duty and retired. I had the opportunity to meet brilliant, talented individuals, people who made history. I observed these patients in the fourth, fifth, sixth, seventh and even eighth decade of their lives, and came to understand what kept them healthy, the good lifestyles, the bad ones, and where trouble lurked.

I met my husband, Mike Wilson, the first day of medical school. We were "Gross Anatomy lab partners"—a polite way of saying we shared the same cadaver. We had both decided at a very early age to be physicians and hadn't wavered. In the old fashioned way, we felt medicine was a "calling", not just a job. Mike is an orthopedic surgeon and relies on me to help him with the medical problems of his patients, and he has done a great job with the oh-so-common arthritis and musculoskeletal problems of my patients. These books are the result of our long collaboration. Married in 1973 while in medical school, we celebrated our thirtieth anniversary in 2003. Our life together has been fascinating and rewarding, and our medical practices have benefited tremendously from our partnership. Throughout this book, Mike has helped me with the medical stories, particularly from his surgical perspective and has been generous with his wit and story telling.

So Let's Join Forces

The husband with his medical risks is my patient and I do everything in my power to prevent a catastrophe. But you can't always get your husband to go to the doctor. If he does go, he is likely to say he has nothing wrong. If he does have something wrong, he may not know it. That is why I am asking you to learn what you really need to know about keeping him healthy.

CHARLIE'S DILEMMA

Charlie and Sharon stop at the bookstore on Saturday afternoon. Called "Chuck" as a kid, he morphed into "Charles" in college during his bearded hippie days, and is now back to "Charlie." He is the fifty-three-year-old vice-president of marketing in a small company that was doing well—at least it was doing well until the last few years. The upcoming year looks bad for his business.

As Charlie browses, he notices a best-selling book on cholesterol. Driven by a vague guilt, he pages through it. He thinks about his own cholesterol, which he hasn't had checked in years because he has been too busy to see a doctor. (He doesn't even have a doctor.) He is concerned because his father had his first heart attack at age fifty-seven, just four years older than Charlie is now. (Charlie already has an ulcerated plaque in the primary artery supplying blood to his left ventricle (main heart pump). If that plaque ruptures, he may well die from a heart attack as he sits in a traffic jam. But he doesn't know that.)

As he moves on to the fitness section, he sees his reflection in the window, the twenty extra pounds he carries around his waist and his thinning, graying hair. His image contrasts not so favorably with the guy on the front page of *Men's Health Magazine*—that same guy with the six-pack abs, the black wavy hair and the dumb grin who seems to be on the cover of every fitness magazine these days. Charlie wonders whether he's ever known a guy that actually looks like that. Charlie has let himself go since he starred as a forward on his high school basketball team. He buys an exercise book promising fitness for life, and goes over to the coffee bar to wait for his wife. He is uneasy about drinking coffee this late in the afternoon because he sometimes has trouble sleeping. Hell, he *always* has trouble sleeping; it's just that the coffee makes it worse. The pastries look tempting, but he wonders if he should eat one since it will only add to his expanding waistline.

Charlie's left knee aches sometimes from an old high school injury and his lower back annoys him as he sits through meetings at work. He knows he needs to start working out again. Starting yet another exercise program is like Mark Twain's line about stopping smoking: it's easy; he's done it a hundred times. But this time, he worries that these aches and pains could get out of hand. He doesn't want to see the doctor first, because the doctor might suggest surgery and he can't even consider surgery now because he doesn't have the time to recuperate. He would like to get back into shape, but a co-worker recently signed up with an aggressive personal trainer and was in bed for two weeks with sciatica. Who needs that?

Sharon has a nervous feeling when she thinks of the twenty-five-year-old single mother recently hired as an assistant in her husband's office. (Charlie has had lunch with this assistant recently to listen to her problems and "help" her. But Sharon doesn't know that.) Sharon knows that she herself has qualities of character, experience and strength that a younger woman lacks, but she knows men aren't necessarily scouting for character, experience or strength when moved by their natural desires.

Charlie won't go to the doctor. When Sharon asks him to, he says that he doesn't know what the doctor is going to say and just doesn't want to hear it. He says he doesn't have time. The last time he went to a doctor he had to wait an hour and a half and then he got a pat on the back. It wasn't worth the time or money.

Sharon and Charlie are pulling together right now, stressed by finances and the duty and obligation imposed by every day's demands. Sometimes he is moody and irritable over nothing. But Charlie's wife is trying to love him and figure him out.

REGRETS
AND
LONGINGS

Falling Off the Track

You may wonder why an internal medicine doctor would write about mental health. Isn't this the purview of a psychologist or a psychiatrist? Well, many men would rather tell their regular doctor about their emotional concerns because they still feel stigmatized by seeing a mental health professional. Also, mental health visits to a psychiatrist or psychologist are not a covered benefit in many HMO's, or appointments to that type of specialist may be only partly paid and limited to a few sessions to get the patient back on his feet.

The Simple Version

There is a difference between falling off the track and depression. Falling off the track means the bad things that happen to people and change their lives. Depression may be one of the emotional consequences.

The Details

When I was a doctor in the Air Force, I had the privilege of knowing Major General Tom Rew, the B-52 pilot who led the Linebacker II bombing mission in North Vietnam to end the Vietnam War. He told me the story of the campaign. "Two single files of over one hundred mighty B-52 bombers, one group from a U.S. base in Thailand and the other from a base in Guam met and, within 30 seconds, we fell into formation with our lights out to avoid enemy detection. Heavy clouds often covered North Vietnam. As I flew first in line over enemy territory, I saw the surface-to-air missiles coming at me through the clouds, like Roman candles. I could tell if a missile had locked onto me by the way it stayed in the same position in my windshield. If the missile moved to one side, it had passed me by."

Often I have thought of General Rew's vivid description of

this mission as a metaphor of life. Sometimes we have to fly deep into enemy territory. Sometimes the missiles lock onto us. Sometimes we are shot down. Sometimes we still survive.

This happened to me. After I trained at Mayo Clinic, my dream was to return home to Iowa and serve people in a small town, just as my great-uncle, Dr. Ernest Stumme, had in Denver, Iowa. At the time I was in solo practice. The intensity of that practice is hard for me to imagine, even now. I was on-call seven days a week, and specialists were often one hundred miles away. Our technology and biomedically engineered drugs were far less sophisticated than they are now. A farmer might come in from the field, tell me he had "gas on my stomach," and I would find that he had a cancer that would kill him with certainty in a few months. I had to make those calls alone. Mental illness was not scarce, although the population often did not understand or acknowledge it, and anti-depressants without major side effects had yet to be invented.

After five years in Iowa, something bad happened to me. I enabled a husband to get an appointment for his wife with our group of orthopedists on a today-basis because of her ankle sprain. Over six weeks later, in an unrelated event, the woman died of neurosurgical complications after an aneurysm in her brain ruptured. I was not her doctor, nor was I involved in the diagnosis or treatment of her brain aneurysm. My first knowledge of her demise came when I saw her obituary in our local newspaper. Two years later, I was served with a lawsuit saying that I had caused this to happen on the day I helped her husband get her the appointment for the ankle sprain. Nothing so absurd, unpredictable, or hurtful had ever happened to me.

I learned a valuable lesson from that experience. I cannot see every hit coming, I have to dodge the bullets just like everyone else, and life or other people may do things that I cannot control.

So I moved on to the Air Force as an officer in the medical core. My first commanding officer was the smartest doctor I have ever known. At the first conference I attended with him, he spoke of Black Water fever (malaria of the brain) and of the intricate immune mechanisms that made one patient's gonorrhea infection confined and another's disseminate to the joints and skin. As a doctor in his medicine section, I had to study all the time so as not to seem ignorant. That was the cure for my derailment back in 1985.

Falling off the tracks is not an uncommon phenomenon among my midlife patients. Many go through a time when their lives fall to pieces. In my medical practice, I have observed that a husband's derailment falls into three major categories: 1) an affair, 2) the unexpected loss of a job and 3) chemical dependency.

Coping with, Healing from, and Forgiving Affairs
Affairs happen. The situation is all too familiar. She is attracted to him because he has a good income and has already established himself as a successful husband. He gets involved, usually with destructive consequences to his job, his family, and his emotional stability. When the wife finds out about an affair, and she usually does, it devastates her, particularly if she does not have some secrets of her own. If the man divorces his wife, and leaves her and the children, the amount of money he actually has when his payments to his last family are subtracted, amounts to far less worldly goods than the second wife had anticipated. His retirement date will be postponed for a long time.

Theories abound as to why this happens. A man may long to be eighteen—young, attractive, and free with a choice of mates before him. He may see in the other woman his "shadow", that half of his life he gave up to become who he is and achieve what he has at midlife. He may be seeking wholeness in the image of a woman onto whom he projects his deepest, heartfelt desire; it is not the woman so much as his own need (his animus) reaching out. And marriages do grow stale as people take each other for granted and stop being polite at home. The wife may grow irritable from stress and perimenopause. Sometimes being loved is being known, and his wife has stopped listening to him, or hasn't caught on to his emotional changes, and no longer knows him. A last theory is that some men may have been sexually repressed. Pornography is now so readily available that they start thinking about what they missed, or what they think other people do, even if it is not realistic, and this leads them to do something that they later regret.

A husband came in with a sense of shame last year, telling me his wife requested that he be tested for all venereal diseases and HIV infection. She had discovered that a female employee in his work place had turned his head and that their attraction had been consummated. This man did not love his colleague, he really loved his wife and the life they had together. He did not even know why he had let this happen. He also feared a sexual harassment lawsuit. (As I understand it, no matter who instigates the affair or how consensual it is, the person who has more power and income in the job situation is presumed to have victimized the other party.) I encouraged this married couple to go into counseling together. Since then, I have talked to them both, and they are happy again.

My midlife patients frequently have love affair problems. They may want to get out of the affair, but cannot because of blackmail. ("I will tell your husband." "I will send your wife your emails."). They may have had an affair, regretted it, and now worry that they have picked up a disease. HIV has ratcheted up the fear of consequences of sex. Unhappiness often follows when a person decides to divorce their spouse of many years and marry a "newer model." One of the most cogent descriptions of how an older man feels after having married someone many years his junior, after his older wife "thickened", is in Tom Wolfe's book, *A Man in Full*. His protagonist, in his fifties, turns over in bed one night and thinks, "Who is this woman?" when he sees his twenty-five-year-old second wife lying there instead of his wife of thirty years. He misses his "real" wife.

If a midlife individual suffers a self-esteem injury such as the loss of a job, he or she becomes even more vulnerable to someone outside the marriage. Sometimes married people have an affair just because they feel so heavy-laden in their daily responsible lives and want to feel free. Some men lose desire for their wives, or women for their husbands, because the person they married stops taking care of themselves and puts on weight. Men may seek an affair because the normal decrease in potency as they age alarms them, making them willing to pay any price to recover their waning vigor. I believe that Viagra can prevent this particular destructive factor in long-term marriages, and suggest to my male patients that they take it, even if just to try it.

I treat the aggrieved party, i.e. the spouse who did not have the affair, with anti-depressants to try to stop the plunging lows. A wife will often agonize over the affair, having the vision of her beloved spouse coupling with The Other foremost in her mind. I can make the obsession stop with anti-depressants. The injured party also needs a dose of self-esteem, the courage to go on, and the strength to take care of her children and job. She may need to see her way clear to win back her husband, to find a future without him, or to forgive him.

I also try to get the couple to marriage counseling. If the erring party will not go, I at least encourage the wronged spouse to enter marriage counseling since it can still be effective, even if done with just one-half of a couple. A forty-eight-year-old woman made an appointment with me because her husband and the father of her children, with whom she had lived in harmony for twenty-four years, came home one day and announced that he was leaving her for a bartender he had recently met. He was not kidding. He left and married the bartender.

My patient was devastated at first. I sent her to one of our finest counselors and she worked through her feelings toward her ex-husband and the marriage. With great courage, she forgave him, took stock of what had been good, and decided that she too had outlived the benefits of her marriage. She worked with her children to help them through the trauma. Two years after this happened, her former husband died. He was not my patient but I presume he had a heart attack. She attended the funeral for the sake of her children, and then returned to home and work. I was glad her emotional pain had been resolved, because with her ex now dead, her bad feelings could have always stayed with her.

The argument for counseling one party in a failing marriage, even when the spouse refuses, goes like this. In Chaos Theory, the flap of a butterfly wing in Hong Kong can cause a hurricane in Florida. So many things in life happen as a series of events, actions and reactions that begin with a minute, innocuous and unnoticeable movement. Therefore, small but significant changes, although initially one-sided, may be able to turn around a marriage in trouble as the other spouse reacts to a little kindness, appreciation, or encouragement that things could get better.

Current thinking is that a marriage (unless cursed with spousal abuse, intractable alcohol or drug abuse, or compulsive sexual affairs) deserves a chance of preservation. Married people are usually healthier than unmarried.

Marriages have good times and bad. It is not the time to call it quits when the partners have drifted away as part of the natural ebb and flow of relationships. Just call it drift, reexamine the union and try to save it. Most married couples do not realize the immense value of their marriage until they have unthinkingly jeopardized it. If you find yourself with a marriage counselor who has outdated ideas and encourages divorce, you are probably wasting your time and money.

If the patient I am seeing is the one who had the affair, and whose spouse is furious at him or her, I advise these steps. First, agree to go to marriage counseling. Second, tell your spouse that you will never again have an affair, and mean it. Third, tell the truth at all times and mindfully monitor everything you are saying for truthful content. Fourth, do more around the house. These actions show that, symbolically, you are trying to put the home back together. The betrayed person must be made to feel safe and loved again.

It takes approximately two years to get over an affair, although the anguish dissipates within several months. Relapses of anger and mistrust are to be expected, however. A dream or a hang-up call can precipitate these relapses. The person seeking forgiveness may despair and want to throw in the towel if he or she is convinced that healing should be over with quickly, and that one-step backward means the rapprochement is failing. If both spouses are committed to the marriage, this event in their lives together can precipitate reflection and a richer relationship in the future.

One patient whose husband had an affair resolved her anger and admitted that maybe she had been part of the problem. In counseling, she realized that she had always accepted what her husband said as being what he meant. When they first married, he had said that he did not think sex was a "spectator sport," meaning that more than a little variation was undesirable to him. Twenty years passed while she kept a lid on her creative ideas for sex because that was what she thought he wanted. But during those twenty years, he had changed his mind. Unfortunately, he did not tell her this, and she did not ask. He had also told her that he never wanted her to "whine about finances" because his Depression-era parents had been obsessed with their pennies. So, she managed their money, bought and remodeled a beautiful, large house, paid the bills, borrowed and repaid as necessary, and did not "trouble" him about money. What he did not mention, however, was that since he had grown up as a poor boy, he felt out of control when it came to borrowing any money. Even if she was doing an excellent job of investing for them, it made him feel insignificant. Marriage counseling forced them to talk about sex, money and power. Since then, their lives have become richer and their roles less restricted. Their sex has become lot more fun, according to her, and he is happy to know that he is a rich man when all the money is counted.

If the errant spouse is a chronic philanderer, that is a different situation. Sometimes the wife chooses to stay with him because she does not see that she has other options, and sometimes the marriage must end because the philanderer has intractable narcissistic characteristics. One woman attempted suicide when she finally acknowledged that her husband was not, nor could ever be, the person she thought she knew. They went into counseling where she found that she would be better off without him.

Loss of Employment
Another cause of falling off the tracks is the loss of a job after a number of years. A company may downsize or ruthlessly let a midlife employee go because his skills have become obsolete, or because they have decided to hire a cheaper, newly educated worker. Loss of a job can precipitate depression. This is another time when I suggest anti-

depressants for several months. I also counsel my patients on how to prevent a tailspin in situations like this. A person should always keep several hobbies and options in mind that could expand into another career. Sometimes the next career can be even more lucrative and fun than the previous one. The old saying, "Out of the ashes rises the Phoenix" certainly applies in this situation.

One man had worked at the same oil company for seventeen years. He was competent and had expected to retire with the company. When the company consolidated and moved to a new location, they abruptly eliminated his job, leaving him to wonder what he was going to do with the rest of his life. He had always been artistic. With the help of anti-depressants and counseling, he decided that he would go back to the university for a Master's degree in Fine Arts. He is doing well, and I believe he will be able to follow this new dream into the next phase of his life.

I also encourage all my patients to acquire computer skills and keep them current, as they are very necessary in today's workplace. If you have to apply for another job, even temporarily, you cannot compete without computer knowledge.

Chemical Dependency
A separate chapter is devoted to the important topic of alcoholism.

And....the road to Hell is paved with good intentions. (I am talking about how easily a patient can become addicted to prescription drugs such as narcotics, tranquilizers, and sleeping pills.) Every doctor probably has a story like this, but I will tell you my story that will always haunt me. An intelligent patient chose me for his doctor. He would leave me messages, preferring not to talk personally, at first asking me to call in a few sleeping tablets for jetlag during a trip, or pain pills for his killer headaches, or Xanax for situational stress at work. I wanted to help him in each situation so I did not say "no" to him, nor question him about the need for these medicines because he always had a logical explanation. I was a little more lenient than I should have been, and I was careful to prescribe a finite amount of medicine. I made small decisions, each of which could have easily been made the same way by a righteous person. But in the end, it was harmful to my patient. Later I found out that I was not the only doctor prescribing medicine for him and he was addicted to prescription medicines. He had managed his addiction by outwitting doctors, almost like he would play a game to win. Unfortunately, he lost his job, and it was a long road back to recovery.

Not Everything That Happens to You Has to Be Good

I learned something important about just living through the hard times when I left my private practice in Iowa. I was in despair, racked with anger over the crazy legal problems that seemed so unjust. Shortly after I began practicing medicine in the Air Force, Lt. General Jack Flynn spoke to the doctors. He is the highest-ranking pilot to have been shot down and captured in North Vietnam, and he spent close to six years as a POW in Hanoi, enduring unspeakable things. When he was released, thin and worn, he was flown to Clark Air Force Base in the Philippines. Because of his rank he was first to call home. He phoned his wife and said, "Mary Margaret, this is Jack Flynn." She said, "Jack Flynn, where have you been?" He told us, "The humor in her voice told me I would be all right." He also said, "When I heard the thunder of the B-52's in Linebacker II, I knew they had come to take me home."

General Flynn did not regret his years as a POW. He said, "If you can accept that not everything that happens to you is going to be good, then you can enjoy a broad range of human experience."

Falling into Darkness:
Depression in Men

The Simple Version

If your husband is angry and irritable, he may be depressed and not know this.

The Details

Real men don't eat quiche or acknowledge depression. The word "depression" is simply not in their vocabulary. In fact, they will rarely initiate a discussion of their moods, preferring to dance around the edges of the subject. When questioned directly they may admit to all the symptoms—sleep disturbance, sadness, and loss of interest in things that usually bring pleasure—but they just will not use the D-word. Men feel it is weak or even shameful to be depressed and so they substitute some different nomenclature, such as "stressed" or "down" or "the blues." Women get depression; men get angry.

A man came to me for consultation this past month. I was the tenth doctor he had seen for abdominal pain. My colleagues had already done every appropriate diagnostic test and prescribed most of the remedies I usually have up my sleeve. I asked him if anything had happened about the time the pain started. He told me that six months previously, about the same time his symptoms began, his beloved wife was diagnosed with stomach cancer. She had died a few months later. The love of his life was here one day and gone the next—and so was his joy. Since there was nothing organically wrong with him, I think he had symbolically internalized her cancer and that his emotional pain perpetuated his symptoms. His depression expressed itself as what we call a "somatic symptom."

Cultural Pressures on Men

Humans are the composite of our ancestral genes, modified over millions of years. These genes adapted us physically and mentally and in the process of natural selection, the strongest survived. We are the progeny of those survivors. Ask yourself what it would have taken to survive when the first naked humans left the forest for the savannah, stood upright, and competed with the other large animals. Some members of those first primitive human groups had to compete for resources, guard the tribes' territory, and protect the members of the tribe, and it wasn't easy work. The young men have always been the physically strongest among us. So we can speculate they were chosen for the duty. They could not go alone or they would be killed so they had to go in groups. If one member expressed fear, that fear could be contagious and the whole group would be weakened. What's more, if the hunting group was not successful, the women and children would not get food and the whole troop would not survive. Pair-bonding species also traditionally compete for mates, so the men must appear tough, strong and capable.

Thus, masculine culture, not just in the United States or the last hundred years, but over millions of years, has had adaptation pressure to glorify physical toughness, adrenalin rushes, and suppress vulnerability, fear and pain. Women may wonder why men are not more in touch with their emotions but there is a long biological and cultural history to this.

Before a man can preserve his species, he must first become a man. The struggle begins in the womb where all embryos are originally female but differentiate into male in just fewer than 50% of fetuses. To become a boy in our culture, you must not be a girl. Thus, a boy is pressured to "Cut the apron strings," "Be a big boy" and "Stop crying." The one emotion he is allowed is anger, so anger and aggression are substituted for less acceptable emotions such as sadness or shame.

Disconnection from internal emotions is frequently at the root of masculine depression. If you do not know you are depressed—or if you don't even have a language that includes the concept of depression—then it is hard to do anything about it.

Physical Brain Changes in Midlife That Have Profound Implications for the Better

I will add one more layer of complexity. We know that boys' nervous systems mature more slowly than girls'. They develop the language of emotion later and are less able to cope with psychological trauma early in life. Even physical trauma such as falling on one's head off a jungle gym or having a fever of 105 degrees may be more neurologically damaging to young boys than to girls.

But men's neurological systems catch up with women's and may surpass them. Men change from who they are in early adulthood into a more complex, feeling person by the time they are in their forties. Brain wiring connections continue to increase in men until it is greatest at age 55. (Brain connections start to decrease in women at menopause.) That translates into more thinking and feeling.

The old theory was that a person was well formed by the time he was three years old, so he was stuck with the early negative parental influences and could only live out that predetermined environmental and genetic heritage. Doctors no longer believe in this scenario. Although it is difficult to prove some of these theories without instant autopsies or far more sophisticated PET scanners to record thought processes, doctors presently believe that the brain lays down tracts, which atrophy when no longer used. A specific example is the two semesters of calculus I took in college. I could not sit down and work an equation now because that tract is no longer functioning. It has been replaced by hypertrophied tracts that focus on people's medical problems.

The implication of this idea is profound. It means that people grow and change into mid-age, for better or worse. A person can get over a bad habit. He can learn to love, even if that did not come easily in younger years. He can learn to be giving or peaceful or positive, even if his parents are cold, mean, depressed people. It also hands him personal responsibility. He allows the positive tracts to be exercised and extinguishes the flow through the tracts that are unhealthy or useless. Perhaps this explains why people who have a long, happy marriage seem so much better adapted mentally and physically later in life. They negatively reinforce the unhealthy thought patterns and bring out the best ones in each other.

How These Brain Changes May Affect a Marriage

What I have to say next is something many people do not realize or think about but I see it in couples. A woman may be highly involved in observing her peri-menopausal symptoms and not think her irritability at home is causing a problem. She assumes her husband is the same stoic person she married twenty years ago because she does not know about the physical changes in his brain during midlife. But because the man's brain is becoming more sophisticated, he may just be discovering emotions that were previously hidden from him. He is suddenly reaching out for empathy and someone who is willing to understand him.

This disconnection between couples, and their modified expectations of one another, can cause significant marital drift. When I see this, I usually tell the woman exactly that; that she cannot take her husband for granted, nor assume he has not changed and deepened over the last few years. She needs to find balance between focusing on her own problems and hormonal changes, and being more open to the evolution of she and her husband as a couple. A man may have spiritual needs that were previously unattended and his wife needs to accept these changes. If there is any one word that is most healing, it is "accepting" instead of judging; accepting the people to whom you are closest for who they are and for what they are feeling. Be merciful. Be forgiving. It won't hurt you.

How Being a Father and Son May Affect a Man

Depression and unease may follow when a man becomes a father. Soon after the birth of his first child, a man may experience emotional pain because of the loss of the relationship with his wife. The wife must now divide her attention between her husband and the new child, so she will be tired and less sexually available.

Men may also feel that they are not measuring up as a father causing a gap between who they want to be and who they are. They may experience shame over these ambivalent feelings toward their sons, feelings they may only be able to process later in their forties when they have the time and the resources.

Similarly, in his forties a man may find that his relationship with his own father becomes more ambivalent as his father declines mentally and physically. This experience will be more intense if none of the antagonistic feelings between father and son were ever acknowledged or resolved.

How Depression Manifests in Men

Psychologists and psychiatrists label a patient with a diagnosis of depression according to the DSM<u>IV</u>, a manual listing the criteria for psychiatric diseases. The patient must meet a certain number of these criteria to get a diagnosis. Conversely, if a patient doesn't have a DSM<u>IV</u> diagnosis, the mental health care giver will not be reimbursed by the insurance company. Because men's depression can be so atypical, it is often misdiagnosed and mislabeled. There is no room for nuance such as depression getting better, or depression on a good day instead of a bad one; or a personality disorder under better peer influence with more acceptable behavior. Also, these rigid diagnostic categories do not allow for the growth that may take place at midlife. If a man is diagnosed as depressed or narcissicistic, he may need to be re-evaluated after a year to see if this label still applies.

Anhedonia

Depression in men often causes anhedonia, loss of pleasure in daily activities, food, or sex. A person suffering from anhedonia will sleep less soundly, be filled with a sense of indefinable longing, and may even start to have thoughts about his own death.

I knew a brilliant forty-five-year-old computer analyst who was respected by his coworkers but troubled by a chronic illness that had started seven years before and intractable family problems. He did not reach out and say he was depressed. He just quietly kept trying to do the next right thing as more disappointments piled up in his joyless life. He put all his affairs in order so that his family was well taken care of, then he shot himself.

Chemical Dependency

Psychologists who treated trauma and those who treated chemical dependency used to be in different subspecialties, but now they are coming closer together. Men have a tendency to deal with depression and old traumas with alcohol or other chemicals. Chemical dependency exacerbates depression because it causes unpleasant emotional and behavioral changes in the addicted person. Alcohol—which is itself a depressant—is the common, socially acceptable way of self-medicating stress and depression. The problem is, it's like pouring gasoline on a fire.

Sexual Acting Out

Sexual acting out may be an expression of male depression. The man may feel ashamed of events in his life, such as a job loss when his company consolidates. He knows that, according to the male code, he is not allowed to acknowledge shame. Usually, he will not cope with these feelings by concluding that he is depressed. He may concede that his life is "just not right" and feel that "something" is missing. He may look at his wife of 20 years, who has aged a bit and put on more pounds than she would like, and decide he no longer loves her. He may project his negative feelings about himself onto her to rid himself of unwanted self-criticism. An affair may temporarily raise his endorphins.

This is the common scenario when the married couple comes to joint marital counseling as a consequence of these events. The man is often diagnosed with a narcissistic personality disorder because his actions seemed to disregard the feelings of his family. This diagnosis carries the connotation of incurable incorrigibility. Beware if the marriage counselor seems too hasty in diagnosing and labeling the problem, or declares too early on that the marriage is a goner.

Midlife Crisis

Another cause of depression is the midlife crisis. Up until his 40's, a man may remain emotionally repressed. Then two things happen. First, he is successful enough that he does not have to devote all of his time to "defending his castle and occupying more land." He also realizes that he wants more pleasure out of life, in other words, to be valued and loved. By age 40 he thinks he will soon be old and that his body and energy may deteriorate before he gets his share of fun out of life. He realizes that he has practiced self-denial for too long only to receive very little emotional payoff. He feels the need to seek gratification before it is too late.

He may never have spoken to his wife about his inner

feelings because that would have challenged his concept of masculinity. It is even more difficult for him to share these emerging concerns with her now.

At this age a man may also suffer an emotional shock if he loses a family member or friend to illness, particularly if the deceased is someone his own age or younger. If this is the first time he has had to face his mortality, he may feel shaken by the experience.

This man needs counseling to sort through his priorities, look back on his life's path and accomplishments, and formulate new goals for the second half of his life. Often he has a profound emotional disconnectedness and it is essential that he make an effort to connect emotionally with his family and friends, rather than just working harder. Sometimes he needs to be taught how to have fun. He might need anti-depressants, especially if he has suffered a big loss such as his wife and family through divorce.

Success has a peculiar connection to midlife depression in men. Often a man has achieved inspite of early childhood obstacles, only to feel empty as he gets into his forties because he never dealt with his early difficult feelings of rejection, shame or sadness. Sometimes he symbolically reaches out for something he feels he should have had earlier in life. I saw one such patient reach out and grab a nurse when he came to the clinic for a blood pressure check. This behavior was completely out of character for this staid professional man. He did not realize that it represented the distress of his soul, only that he had a need welling up inside of him.

Non-Medicinal Ways to Treat Depression
Massage, meditation, communing with nature, increasing exercise and taking walks are all tried and true ways to handle gloom. These are physical ways to cope with mind

problems; mind-body medicine is an emerging field that recognizes this and works with these techniques. For the immediate painful episodes such as a fight with your spouse, distraction such as going to a movie is a good way to change the bad mood. In midlife depressions, so often people feel hopelessly stuck in a bad situation. The way out may be a lateral route such as returning to an old interest like music or writing, or learning a new skill like gourmet cooking.

Antidepressant Medicine

Depression is in part an imbalance among the brain chemicals that allow us to maintain a normal mood. Of course, there is interplay between our biology and our environment. Anyone who has gone through depression knows that this is so, but antidepressant medicine can be effective for some people.

Patients usually take anti-depressants for six months to two years, but if the depression relapses, they may need to continue the medicine indefinitely. The problem with anti-depressants, particularly for men, can be their sexual side effects, such as delayed orgasm. Wellbutrin (buproprion, now available in a 40% cheaper generic) is an antidepressant that does not have this side-effect and may actually increase libido.

If mild erectile dysfunction has been part of the concern that precipitated the depression, the use of an antidepressant can be counterproductive. However, this side-effect can often be overcome with Viagra. When I prescribe anti-depressants for men, I am careful to explain to them in advance that there may be sexual side effects that are not intrinsic to the patient, but due to the medicine.

Professional Counseling

Sometimes counseling helps a man with depression, but not always. Some of my patients have worked through earlier traumas, confided secrets to their therapist, and felt much better. I have had other depressed men, who are so out of touch with their own feelings that when the therapist asks them if anything is wrong, they just say, "No, everything is perfect." End of dialogue.

But feelings may be more powerful when they are not acknowledged. A good therapist can make a difference. Psychologists and social workers often specialize in a particular area such as chemical dependency, or teen-age problems, so be sure the counselor takes care of problems like your husband's be it midlife, depression, or marriage issues. If he does not feel he is making any progress with therapy after three months, it is fine to find another therapist who may be more effective. A strong person gets help when they need it.

I referred a forty-two-year-old man for counseling. He had been in the ICU on several occasions for sky-high blood pressure and heart failure. I gave him samples of his medicine so he would not have to pay for it, but he would not take it, even though I begged him. He liked me and listened to me, but only up to a point, even when I told him outright that he would die young if he did not do what I told him to do.

I finally sent him to a psychiatrist. He told the psychiatrist that nothing was wrong and they made no headway. He died at age of forty-six. Each time I saw him, I got the feeling that he was out of place in modern time. A heavy, imposing African American man, he reminded me of an ancient African king who should have been surrounded by gold and hundreds of beautiful wives. However, in present day America, his gambling debts and his inability to feel good about himself had caused him to love life less than he should have.

If you think that your husband may be depressed or out of

touch with pleasure and fun, go with him to the doctor and express your concerns. Or call the doctor in advance of an appointment and tell him that you think your husband may be depressed. Even if a man denies the obvious, there are ways to approach the problem. Someone has to bring it up. If a man is open to counseling, it can be helpful. The most powerful treatment for depression is often the combination of psychotherapy and medication.

Do not ignore the uneasy feeling that death may be stalking him. I have lost a few patients to suicide and I know that death and depression may walk hand in hand. "Behold a pale horse; and his name that sat on him was Death, and Hell followed with him." (Revelations 6:8) Depression can be that rider of a pale horse, but the load can be lightened, and treatment and hope are available.

If you or a loved one is depressed, a useful web site is www.depression-screening.org.

Falling Off the Wagon: Alcoholism

The Simple Version
If your husband is an alcoholic, your life has probably become unmanageable.

The Details

Chemical Dependency
Chemical dependency is a force to be reckoned with. Many of us experimented with mind altering substances in the 60's and 70's and have some sympathy for the politicians caught in the question, "Have you ever....?" Chemical dependency is a brain disease that affects emotions, thinking and behavior. These artificial chemicals substitute for natural neurotransmitters between brain cells such as dopamine. They flood the spaces between the nerve cells so that the normal sense of pleasure is artificially replaced. After awhile, these addicting chemicals change the brain so that pleasure is not experienced except with alcohol or drugs because the normal transmitters that signal pleasure are suppressed. By then, addiction has set in.

During my training at Mayo Clinic, I spent six weeks as a doctor on the Chemical Dependency Unit. Ray I., a wonderful human being and a person in recovery from alcoholism, ran the unit. He taught me about chemical dependency, and that knowledge has been as valuable as any lesson learned in my years of medical practice.

Is Your Husband an Alcoholic?
Alcoholism is technically defined as continued use in spite of physical or psychological damage, inability to control drinking, drinking more for longer periods than one intended, going into withdrawal upon ceasing drinking, becoming increasingly tolerant of the effects, and giving up

important activities in order to drink. In general, anyone imbibing over six drinks a week may be alcoholic, since this amount is considered beyond normal use. The time of heaviest alcohol use is usually from the late teens through the twenties. Up to one third of young male drinkers experience an alcohol-related blackout, a single drunk driving arrest, or fighting when under the influence. This stage of drinking may resolve itself and not go on to become full blown alcoholism, although there are many young adults in Alcoholics Anonymous. Alcoholic's Anonymous www.aa.org has valuable information about alcoholism, including twelve questions you can ask yourself. A person who answers yes to four is alcoholic. I have included these questions here for those of you who do not have Internet access:

Have you ever decided to stop drinking for a week or so, but only lasted for a couple of days?

Do you wish people would mind their own business about your drinking—stop telling you what to do?

Have you ever switched from one kind of drink to another in the hope that this would keep you from getting drunk?

Have you had to have an eye-opener upon awakening during the past year?

Do you envy people who can drink without getting into trouble?

Have you had problems connected with drinking during the past year?

Has your drinking caused trouble at home?

Do you ever try to get "extra" drinks at a party because you do not get enough?

Do you tell yourself you can stop drinking any time you want to, even though you keep getting drunk when you don't mean to?

Have you missed days of work or school because of drinking?

Do you have "blackouts"?

Have you ever felt that your life would be better if you did not drink?

Denial and Alcoholism

Most alcoholics strenuously resist the diagnosis because it means an afflicted person should not be drinking at all. A problem or heavy drinker, or a person who occasionally permits himself to be "over-served," can still make himself believe that all he has to do is take it easy. In other words, he can keep on drinking. To an alcoholic, this may be the most important thing in the world.

Physicians may unwittingly perpetuate an alcoholic's drinking. The patient may ask, "Doctor, do you think I am an alcoholic?" The doctor says something as innocuous as, "Well, you may not be an alcoholic, Mr. Smith, but you sure are drinking too much." The patient will report this conversation at the bar as "The doctor told me I wasn't an alcoholic, but I should drink a little less. Cut me off if I get too much, Charlie."

Only the alcoholic can make the decision as to whether he is alcoholic. Many people now in A.A. have previously been told they were not alcoholic, just under stress or in need of willpower, a change of scenery, more rest, or a few new hobbies in order to straighten out. These same people finally turned to A.A. because they felt, when they were honest with themselves, that alcohol had them licked and that they were ready to try anything that would free them from the compulsion to drink. Some of these men and women went through terrifying experiences with alcohol before they were ready to admit that alcohol was not for them. They stole, lied, cheated, took advantage of their employers, and abused their families. They were unreliable in their relations with others. They wasted their material, mental and spiritual assets. Many others with far less tragic records have turned to A.A. too. They have never been jailed or hospitalized. Their closest relatives and friends may not have noticed their too-heavy drinking. But they knew enough about alcoholism as a progressive illness to be scared. They joined A.A. before they had paid too heavy a price.

A wife sent her forty-seven-year-old husband to see me because she thought he was alcoholic. Their home life had become miserable because he was drunk and irresponsible most of the time. When she yelled at him, he would only drink more and become sullen. This went on day after day, worse on the weekends, and often in front of their teen-age children. His liver tests showed alcoholic hepatitis, a precursor to cirrhosis. I have never seen a patient with alcoholic hepatitis who was not an alcoholic. I told him he was an alcoholic and referred him to a treatment center. There, the doctor took his history and apparently believed the patient's every word, even though the disease of alcoholism is known for its prominent element of denial. The doctor told him he was a problem drinker. The patient latched onto that like salvation, and he has not got sobriety to this day.

Some people may be alcoholic and neither they nor their close ones know it. I have a friend who would never guess himself to be in the throes of an alcohol problem but I am starting to wonder. He has fender-benders, sometimes locks himself out of his house, and more importantly, his relationships often fall apart over words said while drinking. He feels lonely and off-balance. Would these annoyances cease and his relationships improve if he declared himself a teetotaler?

How to Achieve Sobriety

From close personal observation of my patients and friends, and during my twenty-five years of medical practice, I have come to believe that there is no in-between state with alcoholism. Death, pregnancy, and HIV infection are all a yes-or-no proposition, and so is this disease. I no longer believe that problem drinking exists without alcoholism. Only the individual involved can say whether or not alcohol has become an unmanageable problem. If he says that it has, he has accomplished the first step of A.A., acceptance. The healing is then ready to start.

While I was in the Air Force, I had the privilege of knowing and working closely with a retired colonel, John P., in San Antonio, Texas. He had served in Vietnam, and his life later derailed because of alcoholism. He found the strength to get to Alcoholics Anonymous, and he practiced the twelve steps more effectively than anyone else I have ever met. In this chapter, I want to share with you what I learned from Ray I., John P. and other courageous recovering alcoholics I have had the honor to know.

A close friend related his struggle with alcoholism. At an early age he realized he had the genetic makeup of an alcoholic. Alcoholism had occurred in several members of his paternal family, and he knew that he too shared this propensity. His problem began in college with drinking at parties. Since so many of his friends regularly drank to excess, he did not realize that his alcohol intake was excessive or that his intoxicated behavior was unusual. From 1977 until 1991, he would wake up each morning and know that he did not want to drink again. Each evening he would be so compelled by desire for alcohol, that he would have several drinks. In 1991, after a bad incident involving alcohol, he was able to get into recovery through Alcoholics Anonymous and has not had a drink since. The sense of freedom that he now has, since he is no longer beholden to alcohol, is a wondrous thing for him.

My friend did not drink at work; he was not perceived as an alcoholic, and people seldom complained about him. Nonetheless, the chemical had subverted his pleasure principle. Alcohol was such a ready companion that sex with his wife had become a duty that he had to clear up so that he could get on with his drinking because his libido vanished as soon as he started his daily consumption of alcohol. Once he was able to get into recovery, life's pleasures returned to him.

A person worried about his drinking, probably should be. Alcoholics always slip into this addiction without noticing at first. If others, like his boss or family, are worried about his drinking and tell him about their concern that means the addiction has already gone farther than you think, and he is likely to be suffering from the middle stages of alcoholism. Things will only get worse unless he does something about it. Some studies suggest that the average time between realizing there is a problem with alcohol and beginning to do something about it is as much as seven years! By then, a person's alcohol-related problems have almost always worsened. Procrastination and denial are hazardous strategies with which to deal with any disorder.

A highly talented surgeon in the Air Force worked hard, up to twelve hours a day, and had the highest respect of all who knew him. When Desert Storm was declared, he was one of the first to be called up because his superiors believed that his surgical skills would be needed during the coming war. We won Desert Storm with few U.S. casualties so the surgeon had nothing to do for four months but exercise his liver. When he came home from the war, he had developed full-blown alcoholism. He had a disease, probably with a genetic component, given his Irish heritage. He hit rock bottom a few months later, after being picked up on a DWI (driving while intoxicated) charge in an alcoholic blackout, of which he recalls almost nothing. John P. rendered aid swiftly and definitively.

John explained to my friend that alcoholism is not about being drunk; that is just drunkenness. The insanity of alcoholism takes place when the person is completely sober and decides to take the first drink, knowing that it will lead to a pattern of addictive behavior that hurts him and those he loves. John told my friend to remember his last drunk, not his last pleasant drink. My friend has never touched alcohol again and has no desire to. He was so humiliated by his memory of that last Saturday night when he was drunk, that he got acceptance (the A.A. term for accepting that one is an alcoholic) and surrender (willingness to do whatever it takes to get over the disease) within less than twenty-four hours. The Alcoholics Anonymous group also emphasized that not drinking is only part of sobriety. Learning to live life without chemical dependency can be the hardest part of the transition. It requires repairing relationships, making peace with yourself and others, and living one day at a time. This process is called "working the steps." In my opinion, the founders of Alcoholic Anonymous who designed the famous Twelve Steps were responsible for a therapeutic coup equivalent to the invention of penicillin in the twentieth century.

One of my most gratifying cases was that of a fifty-year-old man I met for the first time when he was on my medical service in the intensive care unit, nearly dead from alcoholic liver disease. In withdrawal, confused and agitated, he was deeply jaundiced and I expected him to die. He was married, and his wife still loved him and stuck with him, although she and I both thought the situation was hopeless. He gradually started to get better and became oriented to people, place, and time. Our hospital held a nightly AA meeting. Although he looked as yellow as a pumpkin, he agreed to go. Night after night, he attended those meetings as he became stronger. Two years later, I was surprised at Thanksgiving to receive a dozen red roses. They were a gift from this patient and his wife along with a photograph of them together, taken recently. She was sitting on his lap and both were smiling. The card said simply, "Thank you for giving me my husband's life back."

I see numerous patients who have subtle or not so subtle addictions to alcohol. At times they have ruined their health (cirrhosis, pancreatitis) and their families. Their wives may have left them, or they may have lost their jobs. Often, however, they do not have these overt problems. They just have the daily need to imbibe alcohol. They wish they didn't have this need, but they see no other way to achieve solace at the end of a tough day. Over consumption of alcohol is particularly seductive for many midlife people because most of them have to work so hard and lead lives of heavy obligation. The quick relaxation they get from alcohol seems vital to their ability to carry on the drudgeries of their lives. A number of my patients want to quit and just do not know how.

I address each case in the privacy of my office, explaining to the addicted person that chemical dependency does not just happen to skid row people; it happens to people like us too. Each alcoholic patient gets a book I keep in my office, Living Sober. I buy it for $2.50 through Central Service at Alcoholics Anonymous. I tell the patient that there is no need to return the book to me, and someday they may want to give it to somebody else who needs it. I ask my patient to take vitamins, specifically thiamin, 50 mg twice daily, to prevent Wernicke's encephalopathy, a kind of brain damage that can occur in the acute phase after one stops daily alcohol consumption. Sometimes I give them three days worth of Valium so that they do not have delirium tremens, the old term for withdrawal syndrome. It is hard to predict who will have withdrawal symptoms because patients are often not honest with themselves or me about exactly how much they drink. I clarify that Valium is not a substitute for alcohol, only that I want them to have medicine for withdrawal symptoms if they do take my advice and stop drinking alcohol.

Who Is Going to Have a Particularly Hard Time Getting Sober

My friend, John P., has named the Society of Helpless Spectators of the Descent. By that he means the well-meaning family, friends, and A.A.'s who try to help others recover but are unable to get through to certain persons. An alcoholic only gets recovery when he really wants it. John P. says there is nothing you can do to help someone who does not want help, if they have not had that magical "moment of clarity" that can be hard to predict. Being wealthy is a disadvantage to achieving that insight. Being intelligent is particularly disadvantageous. Being young and healthy is a disadvantage. Being clever or attractive is a disadvantage. Anything that helps alcoholics keep operating in the bizarre half-world to which they have consigned themselves is a delay to recovery. Whether it's at death's door or just by looking in the mirror, a "bottom" is the turning point. Recovery is for those who want it, not those who need it. The good news is that after turning the corner, all those pluses that delayed the bottom become pluses for recovery. It's a strange, strange disease....

Cirrhosis

Cirrhosis is scarring of the liver. Alcohol, a toxin to the liver, causes one-third of cases. In the early stages, a person may have mildly abnormal liver function tests but no noticeable symptoms. As the disease progresses the patient's immune system becomes less effective, the muscles atrophy, and the skin thins and bleeds easily. An alcoholic man becomes feminized with growth of breast tissue and impotence because of an imbalance of hormones. Cirrhosis is irreversible at this stage. As the scar tissue in the liver builds up further, the flow of blood returning to the heart from the abdomen is impeded. The abdomen may swell with fluid called ascites. The patient appears pregnant with abdominal distension. Varicose veins in the esophagus become engorged and may cause vomiting of several quarts of bright red blood. As you might imagine, this is often the beginning of the end even though we offer temporizing treatments.

Planting the Seed

I have had many patients thank me for helping them to recover from chemical dependency. On the other hand, not everyone is able to quit just by having this conversation with his doctor. When I tell a patient how to stop drinking alcohol, I plant the seed, even though I do not know when it will grow. The patient knows that this can remain an open topic between us, and that I am there to help them if they wish to overcome their chemical dependency.

Alcohol is the most common chemical dependency that I see among my midlife patients. They may have experimented with other drugs during college days, but they are not commonly still using them because there is no legal mechanism for obtaining them. We have a good chemical dependency program at Ochsner Clinic Foundation and I refer a patient whose problem is more complicated than I can handle; for example, addiction to prescription painkillers, tranquilizers or illegal drugs.

When I was in the Air Force, I made the following observation. A number of my patients were intellectually gifted people. Some of the older generals, often in their early 70s, drank alcohol daily, even though nobody complained about it or ever thought they were alcoholic. These men would say to me, "Dr. Wilson, why can't I remember as well as I used to?" not thinking that their alcohol consumption was in part to blame. On the other hand, those older generals who didn't drink much, mostly because they didn't care to, were as sharp and bright as they had been in earlier years. Alcohol is a neurotoxin, and kills off precious brain cells. After making these observations, I completely stopped drinking alcohol.

Alcoholism is a common and insidious disease. While it is not something a person can get over by himself, it is treatable. Anyone can locate Alcoholics Anonymous in the white pages of the telephone book, and call to ask them for the nearest meeting place and time. You can bet a group will be closer than you thought, and probably meet sooner than you had hoped. A.A. is free, and they will never be surprised or embarrassed that someone came to a meeting, or by anything that is said there. Getting through the door the first time is the hardest part. Everyone there will have had, or be struggling with, the same kind of problem.

If your husband is alcoholic and can't stop drinking, you can help him by going to Al Anon. It is held in the same places as the AA meetings. Living with an alcoholic spouse makes a wife's life unmanageable. By going to Al Anon, she can learn how not to enable a husband's alcoholism by protecting him from its consequences, and how she can go about getting her own life back in order.

Boot Hill:

How To Prevent Him From Dropping Dead

If He Has Low HDL, You Have A Problem

The Simple Version

A man with low HDL cholesterol is far more apt to have a heart attack by his early 60's. (The HDL is the good kind of cholesterol; it removes plaque from arteries).

The Details

What is HDL Cholesterol?

HDL, a cholesterol carrier, is like the garbage collector of the bloodstream. If plaque is laid down in the blood vessels, the HDL can suck it out of the blood vessel and excrete it in bile. The LDL, (bad kind of cholesterol) deposits cholesterol in a plaque.

Low HDL cholesterol is the commonest inherited cholesterol problem that causes heart attacks in men in their forties and fifties. If I see a relatively young man with heart disease whose father also had heart disease, inevitably his HDL is under 40. Low HDL predicts a heart attack with no other risk factors. Low HDL is more likely to cause a heart attack than high total cholesterol.

I have come to respect a low HDL as a potent risk factor for coronary artery disease. I particularly recall a fit, rugged man whom I saw when he was age 56. His total cholesterol was low at 192, but his HDL level was only 30mg/dl. (The HDL should be at least 35, and preferably over 40.) This man actually had a heart attack right after I completed his physical examination. I believe his low HDL was the cause.

In the following chapters, I will give you more details on cholesterol problems and treatment, but for now, we will focus on a low HDL, one of the scariest problems.

Does He Have Metabolic Syndrome and Low HDL?

You should try to learn your husband's HDL value. This test is usually drawn with a routine cholesterol. If the HDL is less than 45, your husband probably also has elevated triglycerides, another blood fat; a tendency to put on weight around the middle, borderline blood pressure, and one of his parents or his siblings has diabetes. This condition is called metabolic syndrome. It means he has high insulin levels, is overly sensitive to eating carbohydrates, and is prone to early heart disease.

Metabolic syndrome revolves around high insulin levels. Insulin is a hormone made by the pancreas, a gland behind the stomach that is turned on when a person eats carbohydrates. Insulin fills the fat cells when it takes sugar out of the bloodstream. People get into a vicious cycle of more and more weight gain because their insulin levels increase when they overeat and don't exercise, and then store fat more efficiently. This is called hyperinsulinemia, insulin resistance, metabolic syndrome, or syndrome X.

Obesity, inactivity, high insulin levels, high triglycerides, low HDL (protective type of cholesterol), high LDL (harmful kind of cholesterol), high blood pressure, type II diabetes, and hypertension usually group together. (A low HDL and high triglycerides are the most reliable indicator of metabolic syndrome regardless of a person's weight.) Next to smoking, metabolic syndrome is the most important cause of heart attack and stroke.

When this condition is severe, a man may have lowered self-esteem because he can't control his weight. His sexual abilities wane because the fat in the abdomen turns testosterone into estrogen. He may be upset about having to take medicines for several related conditions. He may feel he has lost control of his body and he is often tired and depressed.

What to Do about Low HDL and Metabolic Syndrome

A person can raise his HDL and overcome metabolic syndrome. Even though it is genetic, there are definite environmental factors. The sped up life in this country with lack of exercise and high calorie eating on the run makes it worse. Your husband must literally change his metabolism. The two ways to do this are 45 to 60 minutes of daily aerobic exercise (e.g. on a treadmill, swimming or bicycling), and weight loss with a high protein, low carbohydrate diet. He may not eat sweets, potatoes, bread or rice nor drink sugary drinks like orange juice or sodas because these things cause blood sugar surges.

What His Doctor May Need to Do

His doctor will assess your husband's overall risk for heart disease. Does he have a family history of premature heart attacks? Does he smoke? Does he have high blood pressure? Does he have chest pains, no matter how mild? Does he have inflammation in the lining of his blood vessels measured by a test called a highly sensitive C-reactive protein? Even though your husband may be at a perfect weight, and exercise, he may need cholesterol medicine if he has evidence of heart disease.

Long acting niacin raises the HDL more than any other medicine, but it is not well tolerated because it may cause itching and red skin. Niacin is potentially toxic to the liver, so a liver blood test is done one month after starting it. The statins, like pravastatin, raise HDL just a little, but still have a large effect in preventing heart attacks. Gemfibrozil is another medicine that raises the HDL, lowers triglycerides, prevents heart attacks, and is often used by people with metabolic syndrome.

Raising HDL

Exercise	most effective way your husband can raise his HDL
Stop smoking	helps his health in other ways too
Weight loss	modestly raises HDL
Monosaturated fats like olive oil	raise HDL and heart healthy
Statin drugs	raise HDL by about 5%
Gemfibrozil	raises HDL by about 10-20% and lowers triglycerides
Niacin, a B vitamin	raises HDL by up to 30%

Heart Disease

The Simple Version

If your husband's parents or a sibling have heart disease, he is at risk. Heart disease may not announce itself with any symptoms, just sudden death. Cardiologists are now able to prevent many heart attacks.

The Details

A physician, my partner and friend, aged 44, noticed shortness of breath and fatigue one day when he was running on his treadmill. A few days later, he walked up a ramp to the elevators at Ochsner Clinic Foundation and experienced shortness of breath again. Taking it as a warning sign, he called the Chairman of Cardiology who performed a stress test. His stress test was abnormal. It showed that a large section of the left ventricle, the main pump of the heart, was not getting enough oxygen with exercise, indicating a blocked blood vessel. The cardiologist proceeded with a cardiac catheterization (angiogram) and my friend had a 99% obstruction of the main blood vessel in his heart (the left anterior descending artery). The cardiologist inserted a stent, a cylindrical device to prop open a closing blood vessel, into the narrowed area.

Coronary disease under age sixty is not common and so my friend could have rationalized his symptoms. Although temporarily shaken by this unexpected brush with death, he followed his cardiologist's advice to the letter, and has resumed his practice with the same excellence and verve he had before.

My friend often had dinner with us in the fine restaurants of New Orleans. I observed him to be disciplined about his food intake, always declining dessert, even as I ate every bit of my bread pudding soufflé at the world famous Commander's

Palace in the Garden District. He was in good physical condition and exercised daily.

Why did this happen to him? Weight control and exercise do help to prevent a heart attack, but in his case, he had a genetically adverse lipid profile and a high lipoprotein (a). He also had a recent respiratory infection from chlamydia pneumoniae, a bacterium associated with coronary artery disease because it can inflame the blood vessels.

The treatment for heart disease, stents and cholesterol lowering medicines, are so effective that your husband's chance of dying young from a heart attack is lower than it was twenty years ago. But a heart attack weakens the heart muscle. This chapter discusses the latest thinking on heart disease, what doctors can do to detect coronary artery disease before a heart attack, and options to treat blocked coronary vessels. Most people believe that all you have to know to have a healthy heart is how to eat a low-fat diet, but this assumption has been called into question. As you can see from my friend's near heart attack, it is not that simple.

Defining Coronary Artery Disease and Atherosclerotic Plaque

Heart disease means several different things. What people think of most commonly is coronary artery disease, a blockage in one of the three main blood vessels that supply oxygen to the heart. If such a blockage occurs, it may lead to a heart attack, also called, in doctor lingo, a myocardial infarction. Atherosclerosis is when plaque is laid down in arteries and narrows them. It begins at by age twenty and progresses throughout life. The plaque is composed of cholesterol-laden cells. That is why cholesterol is talked about in the same breath as coronary artery disease.

These atherosclerotic plaques may be stable or unstable. The old thinking was that a blood vessel would gradually narrow, then block off, causing a myocardial infarction. We now see the process differently. The plaque is a dynamic chemical milieu that changes over time. The plaque usually causes no symptoms unless it becomes unstable and ruptures. The ruptured plaque calls platelets to the site, just as they are called to the site of any small cut on the body to stop bleeding. Because a blood vessel is such a small space, the clump of platelets block off the flow of blood. This is called a thrombus. So it is the thrombus that causes the heart attack.

Symptoms of Heart Disease

When I finished my internal medicine residency training, I expected patients with coronary artery disease to complain of angina (i.e., chest pain following exertion, relieved by rest or nitroglycerin tablets). I am a more experienced doctor now, and I do not expect the chest pain to always be typical for this condition. Sudden death with no warning is a common way that men first manifest heart disease. They are more fortunate if they do have warning symptoms. These symptoms may be a discomfort, burning, or pressure in the chest, neck, or shoulders, or shortness of breath with exertion.

This was the case with a sixty-year-old teacher who called me to say that his heartburn was more aggravating. He had tried taking antacids, but without relief. I noted that his mother had died of a heart attack at age sixty-two. Although my patient was a thin non-smoker with well-controlled hypertension and unremarkable cholesterol, I asked him to do a stress test. It was positive. His angiogram showed significant blockage in the three main blood vessels supplying the heart, and he had bypass surgery. He did well with the operation, and has not complained of "heartburn" since.

Sometimes ignoring a symptom can be a fatal mistake. When I was at Mayo Clinic, an esteemed liver specialist, age 55, felt he was having a gallbladder attack (pain in his upper abdomen). He went to his office to wait for it to pass. He did not survive.

Or another scenario. A woman and her husband have a vacation together for the first time in two years. They go swimming in the ocean. Her husband suddenly gets very short of breath. That's the heart attack. That's it.

Symptoms of Coronary Artery Disease

Chest pain, pressure or burning with exertion

Shortness of breath with exertion

Jaw or shoulder pain with exertion

Sudden death without preceding symptoms

Tests for Heart Disease

If a twenty-year-old thinks he has heart disease, he probably does not. Just fearing heart disease does not cause it. After a patient is forty or older, I am more likely to request a stress test for symptoms that could mean coronary artery disease. A simple EKG at rest is not a reliable indicator of heart disease. An EKG stress test is an electrical tracing of the heart while a person exercises, requiring more oxygen and blood flow to the heart. The cardiologist looks for changes in the EKG tracing that typically occur when the heart muscle does not get enough oxygen because the blood vessel supplying it is partially blocked. The cardiologist calculates the maximum level of exercise (called metabolic equivalents or METs, which are multiples of the resting metabolism.) If a person has excellent exercise tolerance his prognosis is good and if he has poor exercise tolerance and also has coronary disease, his prognosis is poor. Doctors also look at the heart rhythm during the stress test. If the rhythm is unstable during or after exercise, it may mean that the person is at risk for sudden death.

A more detailed test, the stress echocardiogram, looks at the movement of the heart muscle with exercise, and may show a portion of the heart muscle is stunned when it does not get enough oxygen. Another way to image the heart muscle with exercise is with a nuclear medicine (radionuclide) stress test. Contrary to the way it sounds, this test involves very little radiation. A very accurate stress MRI is being developed. It works on the same principle: finding the heart muscle that is stunned and under-oxygenated with a faster heart beat during exercise.

If a patient has a positive stress test, we may proceed with a cardiac catheterization. This procedure is done at Ochsner Clinic Foundation up to twenty times a day and has a low complication rate. The cardiologist sedates the patient, numbs the skin over an artery in the groin or arm with lidocaine (the same numbing medicine used in dental offices), and pushes a small wire catheter into the heart. The cardiologist injects dye into the heart blood vessels, takes xrays, and examines the xrays for significant blood vessel blockages. While we use this test all the time, some have questioned its value in the future, since heart attacks usually arise from the rupture of small plaques that are not significantly obstructing a blood vessel. We now have sophisticated CAT scans that give a picture of narrowed blood vessels to the heart. These are not covered by insurance and cost $250.00 at Ochsner Clinic. MRI images of the coronary arteries without exercise (still in the experimental phase) may be even more accurate in showing the soft, vulnerable atherosclerotic plaque.

I use CAT scans of the heart when I suspect someone may have significant heart disease. I recommend the test for asymptomatic people at midlife with low HDL, or mildly elevated cholesterol, or other risk factors for heart disease. If the test confirms coronary artery disease, the patient should probably take cholesterol lowering medicine, and the expense will be worth it. The person with known coronary disease will also be followed more closely by a cardiologist.

I have had a number of patients who benefited from coronary CAT scanning. One was a fifty-two-year-old man in a leadership position, who works at least sixty hours a week and seldom spends much time thinking about his own health. His wife insisted that he make an appointment with me. He claimed to have no chest pain when I questioned him, but I thought he might be the type of person who would not mention it even if he did have symptoms. This man had a history of high cholesterol for which he was taking Lipitor. Reviewing his lab tests, I discovered that his lipoprotein (a), a clot forming kind of bad inherited cholesterol, was the highest I had ever seen. I also thought he might be at risk for a condition known as silent ischemia (reduced blood supply to the heart muscle with no symptoms). He has so much to do and so many people clamoring for his attention, that I doubted he would notice mild chest pain. I had to decide if he had coronary artery disease or just an evil-looking lipid profile so I asked the radiologist to perform a CAT scan. Sure enough, he had bad coronary disease. At cardiac catheterization we found a drop-dead blockage in his main coronary blood vessel and stented it open.

The argument against the utility of this test is that atherosclerotic plaque is a dynamic process. Therefore, the presence or absence of plaque does not predict what it will do, or when it will do it. My argument is that if a person has calcified plaque, it proves that he has had inflammation and cholesterol build-up in his blood vessels in the past, and is at risk for a heart attack. I am not advocating that your husband get this test done immediately, but there are situations where it could be useful. In time this procedure will find its place in predicting the risk of a heart attack.

I am now better able to predict which non-smoking person is at risk for a heart attack before age 70 by using the CAT scan, lipid profile, lipoprotein (a), homocysteine and highly sensitive C-reactive protein level. The paradigm shift in the last twenty years is that doctors try to prevent a heart attack, not just treat it after it happens and the heart muscle is already damaged.

Tests for Coronary Artery Disease

Stress EKG (electrical tracing with exercise)

Stress echo
(ultrasound picture of the heart muscle with exercise)

Stress radionuclide study
(electronic picture of the heart muscle with exercise)

CAT scan of the coronary arteries

Treatment for Obstructed Coronary Arteries

If the cardiologist finds a significant obstruction (over 80%) he may place a stent in the blood vessel to prop it open. If all of a patient's main blood vessels supplying the heart are blocked, then doctors recommend coronary artery bypass surgery. Cardiologists and cardiovascular surgeons devote interest and research to the question of who should have bypass surgery versus the stents via cardiac catheterization. The unresolved concern about bypass surgery is that it triggers a blood clotting (platelet clumping) tendency in the whole body, most importantly the fine blood vessels of the brain. Post-bypass dementia is a feared consequence.

These days, cardiologists stent the blood vessel open after angioplasty; angioplasty is a procedure where a small balloon is distended inside the blood vessel to stretch it open. The blood vessel has a vexing tendency to block again after angioplasty (30-40% restenosis) vs. a lower rate of restenosis (20-30%) with a stent left in place. Sirolimus implanted in the stent, (also called rapamycin), an unusual drug, originally found in a rare bacteria on Easter Island, appears to markedly decrease the risk of restenosis by preventing the growth of scar tissue after a stent. Both the stenting and angioplasty procedures take place during a cardiac catheterization (angiogram), either at the time of the first diagnostic catheterization or when a second procedural catheterization is scheduled the next day or two in the same patient.

A third option other than bypass surgery or angiogram with stent placement, is to use medicine to reduce the angina pain, lower the workload of the heart, and drastically lower cholesterol so the plaque may slowly begin to resorb. Each patient brings a different set of circumstances, so the choice of treatment is individualized.

Options If Your Husband Has Severe Coronary Artery Disease

Cardiac catheterization with stenting to open the artery
Coronary artery bypass surgery

Medicine to lower cholesterol, blood pressure and heart workload, and nitroglycerin tablets under the tongue

Heart Attacks

Most heart attacks happen in patients who have unstable plaque that is not significantly blocking the vessel prior to the heart attack. If your husband has more than 15 minutes of chest discomfort, and doctors think he may have a blocked blood vessel, either by the description of symptoms, EKG findings, or blood tests, the cardiologist will take him immediately to the catheterization lab and open up the blood vessel. Restoring blood flow to the heart muscle is crucial to preventing damage that could later result in heart failure or, in the worst case, death.

Others Common Forms of Heart Disease

Damaged heart valves caused by rheumatic fever are seen less today because antibiotics are used for strep throat. In rheumatic heart disease, the valves through which the blood flowed forward, either leaked, causing backflow with each beat of the heart, or were partially blocked so that the heart had to pump harder.

Mitral valve prolapse is now the commonest cause of a heart murmur in the young and mid-aged, present in 2.4% of the population. There are two forms of mitral valve prolapse. One is probably not actually a disease, and is perhaps over-diagnosed. It shows on an echocardiogram, but does not lead to long-term heart damage. The serious form is more common in men, or patients with MVP in the family, who are older than age 40, and who have a louder heart murmur. MVP causes mitral regurgitation, which is backflow of blood through the heart's mitral valve. Over time, if this condition worsens, the volume overload may dilate the ventricle, the main muscular pump of the heart. A good analogy is to think of a balloon that has been blown up so much that its walls can no longer decompress themselves. We try to find ventricular dilation early and repair the valve surgically. The other problem with backflow through the mitral valve is that it can dilate the atrium, the chamber of the heart that receives oxygenated blood from the lungs and from which the electrical rhythm of the heart originates. If the atrium stretches, the heart rhythm may disorganize, a condition called atrial fibrillation.

Atrial fibrillation feels like palpitations, a fast and irregular heartbeat accompanied by shortness of breath or fatigue. President George Bush had atrial fibrillation when he complained of palpitations while jogging. In his case, it was due to an overactive thyroid. More commonly, this condition is caused by untreated hypertension, obesity, coronary artery disease, or diseased heart valves.

When the heart atrium fibrillates, blood stagnates and may form blood clots. If a blood clot is pumped out of the heart, it goes straight to the brain and causes a stroke. A stroke means that the blood supply, and, thus, oxygen to part of the brain, is cut off. Those brain cells deprived of oxygen die. When this happens, a person may lose the ability to speak, become paralyzed on one side of his body, or lose his vision. To prevent the dreaded complication of stroke, most patients with atrial fibrillation take a powerful blood thinner, Coumadin (warfarin), for a lifetime. Patients periodically have a blood test to check the adequacy of the dose of Coumadin.

Atrial Fibrillation in Summary

Risks for atrial fibrillation:	Hypertension, obesity, over-active thyroid, and diseased heart valves
Symptoms:	Heart palpitations, rapid heart beat and shortness of breath
Most serious consequence:	Stroke

What is my advice to maintain your husband's healthy heart? First, normalize his weight. He must adjust to eating less food in the long-term, avoid sweets, and learn to like fruit, vegetables and lean meat. He should exercise every day, by walking forty-five to sixty minutes outside or on a treadmill, or by swimming or bicycling. He needs his lipid profile (total cholesterol, HDL, LDL, and triglycerides) checked every five years. If they are abnormal, he should work with his doctor to normalize the lipids, even if that means taking cholesterol-lowering medicine. If family members had heart attacks below the age of sixty-five, a lipoprotein (a), homocysteine, and highly sensitive C-reactive protein level may be checked and lowered if high. An angiotensin-converting enzyme-blocking blood pressure pill (ACE inhibitor) is a good choice to lower blood pressure that is consistently higher that 130/85. He should take folic acid to lower the homocysteine and 1000 mg. of omega-3 fatty acids (fish oil) daily. Above all, smoking negates all of the other good things you and your husband may be doing for his health.

Cholesterol: The Good, the Bad and the Deadly

The Simple Version

Total cholesterol is not the key. It just symbolizes many other biochemical actions at the level of the lining of the blood cells. What matters is if he has a heart attack or a stroke.

The Details

Cholesterol is a worry for my midlife patients. Pilots in the Air Force, men afraid of nothing, who had been shot at repeatedly in fighter planes over North Vietnam, or Wild Weasel pilots who dived in aircraft at enemy surface-to-air missiles in order to suppress them, were concerned about their cholesterol.

There is so much information available about cholesterol, but what is true? At Ochsner Clinic Foundation, I have the privilege of working with sophisticated cholesterol doctors in cardiology and endocrinology. With their collaboration I have refined my skills in treating cholesterol (lipid or blood fat) problems in my patients.

High cholesterol tends to correlate with obesity. Since 50 million Americans are obese, there are more lipid problems in recent years. Abnormal lipids are a special problem for immigrants and descendents of people from countries where starvation, not overeating, was a greater risk to life. Some cholesterol is necessary because cholesterol coats most cells in the body and is an important component of hormones.

HDL and LDL

Total cholesterol is usually not the overriding issue. HDL, which is actually a protein carrier of cholesterol, is like the garbage collector of the bloodstream. If plaque is laid down in the blood vessels, the HDL can dissolve it and excrete it in the bile. The LDL, on the other hand, takes cholesterol to the plaque.

What Cholesterol Level Should He Have?

I will summarize the numbers for you. The recommendations were updated in 2001 and are called the New Adult Panel Treatment III risk prevention guidelines. If a person has no other risks for heart disease (such as hypertension, diabetes, smoking, obesity, personal or family history of heart disease), the LDL cholesterol should be less than 160mg/dl and the HDL should be over 40 mg/dl. If more than two risk factors are present, the LDL should be under 130 mg/dl. If diet, weight loss, and exercise do not achieve these goals, treatment with cholesterol lowering drugs is the next step. If a person has diabetes or known heart disease, the LDL should be under 100mg/dl.

Triglycerides are a significant factor in plaque build-up in blood vessels. Old values for normal triglycerides were too high. Triglycerides should be less than 150mg/dl. High triglycerides are caused by eating sweets, drinking excess alcohol, and inheriting an atherogenic lipid profile.

Total Cholesterol

Less than 200	Excellent
200 to 240	Borderline
240 and above	High

HDL (Good Kind, the Higher the Better)

Greater than 60	Best
Between 40 and 60	Not bad
Less than 40	Too low

LDL (Bad Kind, the Lower the Better)

Less than 100	Excellent
Between 100 and 139	Not too bad

LDL (Continued)

Between 139 and 159	Borderline
159 and over	Too high

Triglycerides

Less than 150 mg/dl	Acceptable

The Danger of Inherited Lipoprotein (a)

Although many cholesterol abnormalities are caused by lack of exercise and poor diet, there is a dangerous type of inherited cholesterol called lipoprotein (a). This is a variant of LDL in that it has a "tail", i.e. an apoprotein tacked onto it that causes blood to clot too easily. Coronary artery disease and blood clotting are linked. Some people are born with a high level of lipoprotein (a) that is lifelong. This is a risk factor for heart disease that begins at least 15 years before other cardiovascular risks such as smoking, high blood pressure, obesity and stressful living.

The LDL and HDL do not vary more than threefold among individuals, but blood levels of lipoprotein (a) can range from less than 1mg/dl to greater than 150mg/dl. Thirty mg/dl is the cutoff point for high lipoprotein (a), and a high level is present in 25% of Asian Indians, 15% of Japanese, 15% of Caucasians of European descent and 8% of Hispanics. African-Americans tend to have higher levels of lipoprotein (a), but for reasons not fully understood, it is less toxic in this population.

The lipoprotein (a) level should be tested in patients with a personal history of early coronary disease before age 65, or a family history of sudden death or premature heart disease in their primary relatives (siblings or parents). It should also be tested in adopted people whose family history is unknown, or when coronary artery disease happens in patients with a healthy lifestyle and no other risk factors; and in those who have progression of coronary disease despite stenting, angioplasty, or bypass surgery.

Most doctors do not yet know about lipoprotein (a). I learned about it only last year under sobering circumstances. I have a 56 year-old patient who is an executive engineer in a high-tech company. He is originally from South India and is a vegetarian. This man called me in the fall and told he was experiencing chest pain. My first thought was that this could not possibly be heart disease because he seemed too young, his total cholesterol had always been less than 200, and his diet was ideal, no meat at all. I had him do a stress echocardiogram, but was skeptical of its accuracy when the cardiologist called to tell me it was positive. I apologized to the engineer for being overly cautious, but asked the cardiologist to perform an angiogram. He had severe blockages in all three main blood vessels to the heart. Fortunately, he was able to undergo successful coronary artery bypass surgery the next week.

Later, his friends, who were doctors from India, provided me with medical articles on lipoprotein (a). They were aware of this gene for premature coronary disease in their population. The patients who have the highest lipoprotein (a) levels are those from South India. From that day on I have always checked the lipoprotein (a) levels in my South Asian patients.

The key concept with lipoprotein (a) is that it is only an added danger when the LDL cholesterol is high and other risks for cardiovascular disease are also present.

Homocysteine and Highly Sensitive C-reactive Protein, Other Risk Factors

Homocysteine, an amino acid (part of a protein), is correlated with disease of the arteries. I first learned of this risk factor in conversation with another internist. He told me of a family in his practice where two siblings had strokes in their 20's. This was such a rare occurrence that he sought a genetic explanation and found high homocysteine levels.

An individual's homocysteine level should be less than 10. Five to7% of the population have a higher level that could lead to premature heart attack or stroke.

Just as homocysteine has been in the news this last year, you may have encountered the term, C-reactive protein. Those with the highest C-reactive protein are at risk for heart attack, stroke, and damage to other blood vessels, independent of cholesterol and blood pressure. Doctors order a highly sensitive C-reactive protein and if the test result is higher than normal, the patient may have inflammation in the coronary arteries. Inflammation refers to the action of immune cells, as old as Adam, necessary for human survival against bacteria. To annihilate bacteria, these immune cells have weaponry in the form of toxic biochemicals.

C-reactive protein is not a specific test for heart disease because it is high anytime the body has inflammation, such as a tooth abscess or rheumatoid arthritis. The reason it is associated with cardiovascular disease is that it may represent greater proclivity of inflammatory cells to react in blood vessels and release toxic chemicals. Some have taken this theory a step further and suggested that old chronic infections can over-activate the immune system to the detriment of blood vessels. An example of this is cytomegalovirus (CMV), a virus like mononucleosis. The worst combinations are a low HDL, or a high LDL with a high C-reactive protein indicating an inflamed blood vessel.

Practically, we use C-reactive protein to help us decide if a person with high cholesterol should take cholesterol-lowering medicine, often a lifelong commitment. If the C-reactive protein is in the highest quadrant, doctors are more likely to use medicine to treat the cholesterol. A highly sensitive CRP also helps us in an emergency situation when a patient is having chest pain from heart disease. It signals very high risk, inflammation in not one spot but throughout the coronary blood vessels, and lets us know we must stabilize the patient quickly and aggressively.

What is the role of the bacteria, chlamydia pneumoniae, a respiratory infection that looks like flu in the winter, in blood vessel disease? These bacteria have been found in atherosclerotic plaques and may set off the inflammation that ultimately leads to stroke or heart attack. Some cardiologists and neurologists treat their patients with doxycycline 100 mg. twice daily for two weeks every three to five years to eradicate this infection. The research is not yet available that shows heart attack and stroke may be prevented by treating for chlamydia pneumoniae. This is something to watch in the future.

Global Risk Assessment, Not Cholesterol Alone, Is Important

Global risk assessment means that cholesterol alone does not predict who will have a heart attack. Rather, it is the combination of the risks in the table below that more accurately predict who will have a heart attack or stroke in the next ten years. People with diabetes, poor blood flow to the feet, blocked carotid arteries in the neck, or an abdominal aneurysm have very high risk for associated coronary artery disease, at least a 20% chance of a heart attack or stroke within the next ten years.

Global Cardiovascular Risk Assessment

Total cholesterol

LDL (bad kind of cholesterol that deposits plaque in blood vessels)

HDL (good kind of cholesterol that removes plaque from blood vessels)

Lipoprotein (a), a bad kind of inherited cholesterol

Global Cardiovascular Risk Assessment (Continued)

Homocysteine, may be inherited in high levels causing heart attack or stroke

Highly sensitive C-reactive protein (a measure of inflammation in blood vessels)

Smoking

Diabetes

Hypertension

Carotid artery disease and abdominal aortic aneurysm

High body mass index (truncal obesity) (Go to website www.weightloss-basics.com to calculate his BMI from height in inches and weight in pounds).

At least 20% of cardiovascular risk is determined entirely by family history.

Preventing Coronary Artery Disease: What Your Husband Can Do for Himself

Diet and Exercise

Atherosclerotic plaques can change for the better as good and bad cholesterol ratios shift with weight loss and exercise. A person who loses 10 pounds and does daily aerobic exercises, such as walking, bicycling or running, or aerobic exercise in the gym, raises his HDL (good cholesterol) and lowers his LDL. A pure vegetarian diet may lower the cholesterol about 10 %. If cholesterol can be lowered by diet and exercise, clearly that is the simplest strategy. A dietician's cholesterol advice is at the end of this chapter.

I used to think that cholesterol was a long-term problem that over the years would build up to its destructive potential. Recent studies have shown that a single high fat meal such as a steak may be detrimental in the moment. The fat globules in the blood increase significantly after a high fat meal and may impede blood flow. Ultrasound observation of blood vessels has shown decreased blood flow within a few hours after a high fat meal. Doctors believe that blood flow through the small vessels or capillaries (called the microcirculation) may be impaired by a single high fat meal. The risk of sudden death from an arrhythmia during a heart attack is associated with eating very high fat meals. The problem from one meal may not last more than a few hours but you can extrapolate the effect over many high fat meals. I guess the bottom line is, don't let your husband order a thick steak when he takes you out.

Aerobic Exercise
Exercise capacity has recently been shown to be the most important predictor of whether a person will die from heart disease. The positive effects of daily exercise on the blood vessels, heart muscle, and brain tissue simply cannot be overemphasized.

Aspirin
One coated baby aspirin a day (for example, 81 mg of Ecotrin) prevents platelets from accumulating in one spot causing that fatal thrombus. A recent controversy arose as to whether concomitantly taking a non-steroidal anti-inflammatory medicine such as ibuprofen negated the blood-thinning effect of the baby aspirin. The study that raised the question was not done in people, but in the lab, and looked at only one anti-inflammatory medicine. Presently, we do not believe that taking both cancels the benefits of either although the question is still unresolved. Also, about 5% of people are resistant to the blood thinning effect of aspirin. Presently we do not have an easy test to determine who this is.

Folic Acid
Folic acid is a B vitamin doctors recommend to prevent coronary artery disease and stroke because it lowers homocysteine, a part of a protein that may be toxic to blood

vessels. Folgard and Foltx are prescription combinations of folic acid, B12, and B6. Everyone should get at least 400 micrograms of folic acid daily. Stroke, dementia, and heart attacks may be in part prevented with this vitamin supplement.

Cardiologists recommended antioxidant vitamins in past years, but the research proving benefit from anti-oxidants has been disappointing, so I am presently not recommending vitamin E or C to my patients. Doctors recommended against vitamin A (or beta carotene) supplements when research showed that it increased the risk of lung cancer in smokers. Eating green and yellow vegetables is a better way to get natural anti-oxidants than vitamin pills.

Fish Oil

Fish oil seems to stabilize the heart rhythm and prevent sudden death. It is also a valuable and inexpensive adjunct to prevent and treat atherosclerosis. EPA and DHA are omega-3 (also called long-chain n-3) fatty acids. They should be taken in combination capsules at a dose of 1000 mg a day if your family does not eat two or three fish meals a week. Eskimo and Inuit persons who eat a lot of fatty fish have a low incidence of heart attack and this observation led to the discovery of fish oil as important for the management and prevention of coronary artery disease. The mechanisms by which omega-3 fatty acids slow atherosclerosis are several and complex. They probably work by decreasing inflammation in blood vessels. They may also prevent sudden death by stabilizing the heart's electrical system, particularly in the setting of an acute heart attack. So far, no serious side effects are known that require monitoring and the capsule is not unpleasant.

Fish for a Healthy Heart

Salmon

Fish for a Healthy Heart (Continued)

Atlantic herring

Albacore tuna

Anchovy

Bluefish

Swordfish

Mackerel

Arctic char

Fish Oil Supplement Examples

Super-DHA	(by Carlson 1-850-323-4141)
Super-EPA-500	(by Bronson 1-850-235-3200)
Cardiotabs Omega 3	(by Cardiovascular Consultants 1-850-811-1007)

Smoking

Smoking is the single most damaging thing a person could do to his heart. Even if the cholesterol and blood pressure are perfect, smoking will still damage the blood vessels, at a young age. Cigarette smoke constricts and inflames the blood vessels to the heart, brain, legs and genitals. I have a 48-year-old man whom I have seen for a yearly physical for the last 9 years. He has smoked many years and tells me he does not want to quit. During each exam, I try to feel the pulses in his feet and they are feebler every year. Since atherosclerosis is a whole body disease, I know the same narrowing is taking place in the blood vessels to his heart and brain.

Preventing a Heart Attack

Daily aerobic exercise and maintain fitness

Normalize weight

One coated baby aspirin (81 mg.) daily

Folic acid to lower homocysteine

Preventing a Heart Attack (Continued)

3-omega fish oil, 1000 mg. daily

Stop smoking

Ask the doctor for a lipid profile and compare the results with normal values

What His Doctor May Do to Prevent a Heart Attack

The doctor will try to keep his LDL or bad kind of cholesterol under 130 mg/dl and under 100 mg/dl if he has more than two other risks for heart disease or diabetes. The doctor will maintain the blood pressure under 130/85 with weight control and exercise or blood pressure lowering medicine. Of these, angiotensin converting enzyme (ACE) inhibitors and angiotensin receptor blockers (ARBs) seem to do the most to dilate blood vessels and prevent the biochemical events in vessels that lead to heart attack.

Cholesterol Lowering Medicine

Cholesterol (lipid-lowering) drugs are the answer for many people. Genetics over which we have no control, often determine how much cholesterol, both good and bad, the liver manufactures and these medicines signal the liver to stop manufacturing cholesterol. In the future, combinations of the drugs that lower cholesterol will likely be used more. This allows lower doses of each, fewer side effects, and synergism among them.

Niacin

Niacin is coming back as a treatment for high cholesterol. It is the only medicine that reliably raises HDL up to 30% and lowers lipoprotein (a). So if the patient has a primarily low HDL or a high lipoprotein (a), this is the drug of choice. Doctors cannot give niacin to patients who have diabetes or gout because it may aggravate these conditions, although we are rethinking whether diabetics may use niacin. The red undertones of the skin it causes are not an allergic reaction.

Niacin was reformulated as the prescription drug Niaspan for fewer side effects. Niacin is also available in inexpensive over-the-counter preparations.

HMG CoA-reductase Inhibitors (Statins)

The HMG CoA-reductase inhibitors, also called statins, decrease the level of LDL (bad cholesterol) by blocking the enzyme in the liver (HMG CoA-reductase) that manufactures it. Statins also block the manufacture of the protein that carries cholesterol and triglycerides to atherosclerotic plaques. They increase the sensitivity of the LDL receptors in the liver so the liver more efficiently clears LDL from the blood. Doctors have watched the incidence of heart attack and stroke decline as these remarkable drugs have been available to patients in the last ten years. In my practice, I commonly prescribe Pravachol, Zocor and Lipitor because they are proven to decrease heart attack and stroke. Some of my patients have dropped their LDL cholesterol from over 300 to under 200. This is a substantial decrease and has a major deflating effect on those bloated plaques.

The liver's manufacture of cholesterol peaks at 3 a.m. Therefore, the statins Pravachol and Zocor are given at bedtime so they can be maximally effective when that peak occurs. Lipitor acts over a four day instead of a six hour period so may be given any time during the day. Sometimes it causes insomnia so we move the dose to the morning.

Not only do statins reduce the risk of heart attack, but studies are now showing they also decrease the chance of stroke. Statins do not dissolve plaque according to angiograms done after people have been on them for awhile. Their benefit is derived by decreasing cholesterol in bloated plaque, stabilizing plaque so it is less prone to rupture, preventing blood clot formation, decreasing inflammation in the blood vessels (lowering C reactive protein) and dilating blood vessels to increase blood flow. Early studies suggest that the statins decrease the risk of dementia and boost bone formation, decrease fracture risk in osteoporotic people, and may cut the risk of diabetes. You should watch for more information on benefits of statins outside the cardiovascular system.

Liver toxicity is a potential side-effect of all the HMG CoA-reductase inhibitors and niacin. I monitor my patients for side effects, but liver toxicity only occurs in about 1% of patients. To check for liver toxicity, the patient has another lipid profile a month or two after starting the medicine to document its efficacy, and a liver test called an SPGT. If all is well, these tests can be repeated every six to twelve months. Another side-effect of HMG-CoA-reductase inhibitors is muscle aching. A blood test can be done to check for an elevated muscle enzyme in the blood (CPK). If a patient has generalized muscle aching on statins, we stop the drug. Some of the muscle toxicity is only visible on a muscle biopsy so cannot be detected by the CPK test.

In 2001, a letter in the newspaper from a patient asked whether taking statins worsens memory because he had worse memory and was taking it. We do not know if that side-effect may occur in some, but this group of drugs has been shown to lower the risk of Alzheimer's disease. Statins do interfere with sleep in some patients and poor sleep leads to poor memory.

Lastly, if a patient stops his or her statin when entering the hospital, they may experience a rebound inflammation in the blood vessels and be at increased risk for a heart attack. What bothers me about this is that many of my patients cannot always afford their medicine any given month so they go on and off these drugs. With this information about a possible rebound effect, I caution them to take the cholesterol lowering medicine consistently.

The cholesterol medicine, Baycol (cervistatin), was taken off the market in 2001. The complication of muscles toxicity (rhabdomyolysis) was at least fifty times higher than that side-effect with other cholesterol lowering statins. Nonetheless, this made the news during a relatively dry news spot during the summer so it was talked about over and over in the media. This led some of my patients to throw away their cholesterol pills, an overreaction because we seldom see this side-effect with the other statins. We do tell our patients when they start a statin that they should let us know if they have any muscle aches that seem new.

New potent HMG CoA-reductase inhibitors are being tested now that will drastically lower the LDL. Another drug (called CETP inhibitor which blocks the cholesterol ester transfer protein) raises HDL dramatically and is now in development. Combinations of statins and niacin will be readily available in the next few years. Some statins may be better than others. For example, Pravachol (pravastatin) has twelve or more studies proving it prevents heart attacks even though the actual cholesterol value may not be lowered as much as with other statins. An older statin, Mevacor (lovastatin) is available as a generic and probably works almost as well as the others. It is cheaper than the brand names.

Should Your Husband Take a Statin?
Yes If He Is Over 45 and:

Has heart disease

Has diabetes

Smokes

Has a family history of premature heart disease

Has elevated total cholesterol and LDL cholesterol over 130 and low HDL

Has an elevated LDL and a high C reactive protein

Has a 10% or greater chance of a heart attack in the next ten years

Zetia (Ezetimibe)

This is a new cholesterol medicine that prevents the absorption of cholesterol. It may be added when the statins alone do not achieve sufficiently low cholesterol. The few patients of mine who take it do not seem to have had significant side effects yet. It is too new for any studies that prove it prevents heart attack or stroke and to know the long term side effects. Ezetimibe may be added to a statin when the statin alone does not sufficiently lower cholesterol to safe levels in someone who has known coronary artery disease or is at high risk for getting it.

Gemfibrozil (Lopid)

Some patients have high triglycerides and a low HDL and only a modestly increased or normal LDL (bad cholesterol) level. This pattern holds a high risk for cardiovascular disease (heart attack and stroke), and cardiologists have come to fear it. Well done scientific studies have shown that gemfibrizol (Lopid), 600 mg taken twice daily lowers the triglycerides, raises the HDL, and clearly helps prevent heart attack and stroke. Potential side effects include the same muscle soreness I described above and, possibly, elevated blood sugar.

One of my patients was a retired Air Force officer who had mildly elevated cholesterol, high triglycerides, and a low HDL. We tried all the lipid lowering drugs, Questran (a powder not used much any more because it lowers the HDL), Lipitor, and Lopid. He could not use niacin because of his gout. He and I looked at a lipid profile after he had been on each of the medications for six weeks. His personal best was on gemfibrizol. He is fifteen years older now, and still has not had a heart attack or stroke.

Tricor (fenofibrate) is a newer, more expensive form of a gemfibrizol kind of drug. It may be used to lower triglycerides when that is the primary abnormality.

Lowering Lipoprotein (a)

Lowering the LDL, even without lowering the lipoprotein (a) inhibits progression of coronary lesions, because LDL acts in tandem with lipoprotein (a). The studies showing lowered lipoprotein (a) alone prevents heart attacks and strokes are not yet finished but doctors believe that lowering it will be beneficial. A person cannot lower this bad kind of inherited cholesterol with diet, weight loss or exercise. Niacin and fish oil supplements lower it.

Lowering Homocysteine Levels

Lower homocysteine is not proven to prevent heart attack, stroke, dementia or death, but it has been shown to prevent recurrent blood vessel obstruction in the heart after stents and angioplasties. Await the studies that prove that lowering homocysteine prevents heart attack and stroke. Folic acid supplements lower homocysteine.

Lowering C-reactive Protein

Aspirin is a potent anti-inflammatory. This is one of the prime mechanisms along with its blood thinning properties, by which aspirin prevents heart attacks and strokes. The statins, potent cholesterol lowering drugs, also lower C-reactive protein and decrease inflammation in the blood vessels. Fish oil and treating chlamydia pneumoniae lowers the inflammation in the blood. New research is emerging that 1000 I.U. of vitamin D is anti-inflammatory. Cardiologists now view this inflammation in the blood vessels as the key to precipitating a major stroke or heart attack. Watch this area for further developments.

How to Raise HDL (the Good Cholesterol) Levels

Weight loss

Aerobic exercise

Niacin

How to Raise HDL Levels (Continued)
Statins

Gemfibrizol

How to Lower LDL (the Bad Cholesterol)
Low cholesterol diet

Daily aerobic exercise

Weight loss

Niacin

Statins

How to Lower Lipoprotein (a)
Niacin

Fish oil

The Goals of Cholesterol Therapy
Prevent a heart attack or stroke

Raise HDL

Lower LDL

Lower triglycerides

Lower homocysteine

Lower C-reactive protein and inflammation

Lower lipoprotein (a) or render it inactive by lowering LDL

What to Look for in the Future
A new laboratory test that checks for 21 subtypes of cholesterol, the VAP test, will soon be available and will allow a more targeted risk assessment than total cholesterol levels. Other blood chemistries and perhaps even infections that affect the arteries will be shown to play a role in the development of unstable plaque.

Watch for new combination cholesterol-lowering drugs that

contain a statin and niacin or inhibitor of cholesterol absorption. Also watch for previously unknown side effects of these combinations.

I want you to consider two things when you read about breakthroughs in cholesterol problems. First, it really doesn't matter *what* the cholesterol is. What matters is the endpoint, whether a person has a heart attack or stroke. Drug companies must prove a reduction in cardiovascular events, not just a reduction in cholesterol, before they can claim that their medicine helps people and the long-term expense and potential side effects are worthwhile. Second, you must beware statistics. For example, if a cholesterol drug were given to 100 persons and one had a heart attack, while of the 100 who did not take the drug, two had heart attacks; the pharmaceutical company will tell people they have demonstrated a 100% reduction in heart attacks in those who use their drug. The underlying numbers suggest a different story. Having said this, most middle-aged doctors I know are taking cholesterol-lowering medicine themselves (particularly Pravachol) because of what we presently know of the benefits.

Addendum: A Dietician's Instruction to Lower Cholesterol.

(I put this at the end because if your life is as busy as mine, neither of us have the time to sort through different types of fats daily. It would be nice, but so would a less busy life.)

When patients are instructed in a low cholesterol diet, they learn about different types of fat in food. Animal fats and vegetable oil are both naturally abundant. Saturated fat should be limited. (In organic chemistry, saturated means the backbone of the fatty acid has a carbon bond at each connection.) Saturated fats are found in whole milk, cheese such as cheddar, American and Swiss, butter, cream cheese, sour cream, ice-cream, and heavy cream-based sauces. Land animals' fat is 40-50% saturated compared to vegetable oil that is only 20% saturated. Therefore, patients are advised to have no more than three servings a week of beef or pork (including bacon, pork rinds, and chitttlerlings) and no more than three egg yolks a week. Organ meats like liver and kidney are poor choices, but who eats those anyway? Chocolate made of cocoa and butter is high in saturated fats. Commercially prepared sweets contain eggs and butter and we discourage eating them.

Trans fats in solid margarine and fast food are also unhealthy. Unsaturated fats are healthier; you can identify them because they tend to be liquid or oil at room temperature. (They have a lower number of carbons links in the chain.)

Monounsaturated fat is best for cholesterol lowering. The classic example is olive oil. Foods that also contain monounsaturated fat include canola oil, peanut oil, olives, peanuts, peanut butter, avocados, pecans, almonds, and cashews. My patients are always amazed that they are allowed to eat some nuts. The key is moderating the quantity (i.e. no more than one third cup of nuts). A large quantity of almost any food is fattening and high body fat correlates with high cholesterol.

Polyunsaturated fats lower the LDL but also lower the HDL so are not entirely harmless. Americans tend to over consume them. They should not have more than two servings a day of margarine or salad dressing. Corn, soybean and safflower oil are the polyunsaturated oils on the market that comprise margarine and salad dressing. Walnuts and English nuts contain polyunsaturated fat.

Benecol (also called stanol esthers) is like margarine and tastes about the same. It is made from plants and lowers total cholesterol and LDL by about 10%. The only reason people do not eat this rather than regular margarine and butter is that it is over four times as expensive although it is available in most grocery stores.

My patients may say, "I have a long list of things I am not supposed to eat, but what can I eat? What is healthy?" The diet recommendations, especially for those who want to lose weight, are changing. Results from large numbers of research patients should be available soon. The trend is to lower carbohydrates but get them in the form of five or six servings of fresh fruit (but not fruit juice due to high sugar content) or vegetables daily. If the vegetable is cooked, it should be steamed and still crisp to eat. If carbohydrate intake is lowered, protein and fat will increase in proportion.

Foods That Raise Cholesterol
Whole milk

Butter

Chocolate

Food Containing Monounsaturated Fats That Lower Cholesterol
Olive, canola, and peanut oil

Olives

Avocados

Peanuts, pecans, almonds, and cashews (no more than one-third cup)

Polyunsaturated Fats; No More Than Two Servings a Day
Margarine

Salad dressing

Corn, soybean and safflower oil

Other Cholesterol Lowering Substances
Fish oil (decreases triglycerides by 25-35%)

Soy protein (dose of 20-30 grams/day decreases LDL by 5-7%S)

Other Cholesterol Lowering Substances (Continued)

Stanol esthers (e.g. Benecol substitute for margarine decreases LDL by 10-15%)

Fiber (large doses of over 10 grams/day decreases LDL 1-10%)

Hypertension

The Simple Version

Let me tell you right up front why hypertension matters. If the blood pressure is greater than 130/85 consistently, it will damage brain cells and make a person dull-witted in old age. If mental abilities matter to you, then blood pressure matters to you.

The Details

Normal Blood Pressure

Hypertension does not mean high emotional tension. It is not a mental state, nor is it due to stress. It is a physical condition. If your husband's parents had hypertension he is much more likely to have it. Hypertension is multifactorial, having to do with the "thermostat" in the brainstem that sets the blood pressure, the resistance in the blood vessels (that become stiffer with age) and certain hormones (the critically important angiotensin and renin) secreted by the kidneys, heart and blood vessels. One in four Americans will eventually have hypertension and it is more common as people age.

A normal blood pressure is less than 120/80 and prehypertension is a blood pressure of 120-139/80-89, measured in millimeters of mercury (mm Hg). Blood pressure changes throughout the day and with the level of physical activity. The top number is the systolic pressure generated as the heart beats and the bottom number is the diastolic pressure when the heart relaxes after a heart beat. Both are important and need to be normalized. If the pressure is consistently high, it damages the blood vessels. The analogy is to a pipe that, over a long period of time, is subjected to pressures higher than those for which it was made. Eventually, that pipe becomes corroded. A more apt physical description of the damage is sheer stress. This is stress applied in parallel, as opposed to a head-on collision.

Blood Pressure Categories

Ideal:	less than 120/80
High normal (prehypertension):	130-139/80-89
High:	greater than 140/90
Stage 1 hypertension:	140-159/90-99
Stage 2 hypertension:	160-179/100-109
Stage 3 hypertension:	Greater than 185/110

Why is blood pressure so important? High blood pressure is the main cause of stroke later in life. A person may have one large obvious stroke or multiple small strokes of which no one is aware until he can't walk without falling and can't remember much. High blood pressure also leads to heart attacks by damage to the blood vessels that supply oxygen to the heart muscle, heart failure when the main pump can no longer pump against so much resistance, and disordered heart electrical rhythms called atrial fibrillation. People can develop these diseases even without hypertension, but making the personal choice to take his blood pressure medicine alters the risk in your husband's favor.

So, it is not the high blood pressure itself that is the disease but its effect on target organs including the brain, heart and kidneys. High blood pressure usually causes no symptoms so is called "the silent killer". However, patients often experience subtle symptoms of non-well-being such as fatigue, headache, shortness of breath and sexual dysfunction when they have untreated hypertension. If an echocardiogram (ultrasound of the heart) shows a thickened heart muscle called left ventricular hypertrophy, it means the person with hypertension is more likely to have a heart attack or stroke. Similarly, if the urine contains protein, it means that the kidneys are being damaged by hypertension.

I was the fourth doctor a sixty-year-old man consulted about his hypertension. He came to me because he was looking for a doctor to say he did not have to take medicine to lower his blood pressure. He placed an enormous priority on maintaining full sexual function later in his life. He was concerned that any prescription medicine could limit his abilities. I told the gentleman that we had medicines to treat hypertension that dilate blood vessels and may even improve erectile function. He did not buy my explanation or the medicine I prescribed. He left and did not return. I made several attempts to follow up with him. When I last called his home to encourage him to treat his blood pressure, his wife said she appreciated my efforts in trying to help him, but that his mind was made up. His obituary was in the newspaper one year later. It stated that he died of a stroke.

Causes of Hypertension

Obesity

Genetics

Too much salt in the diet in some but
not all hypertensive patients

Increased resistance in blood vessels from older age

A higher set level of blood pressure determined
by the deep structures of the brain

Less commonly, a blocked renal artery or an adrenalin tumor

Consequences of Long-term Untreated Hypertension

Fatigue, headache

Damage to the eyes, kidneys, and heart

Stroke

How Your Husband Can Lower Blood Pressure

A twenty point drop in blood pressure can cut in half the risk of stroke and heart attack. A 20 lb. weight loss may cause a 20 point drop in blood pressure, exercise may take 4 to 9 points off blood pressure, less alcohol intake may take off another 2 to 4 points, and a low salt diet may help lower blood pressure. If your husband loses ten pounds, even though it might not be the whole twenty-five pounds he would like to lose, he will still lower his blood pressure. Those who drink alcohol every day tend to have hypertension. Alcohol destabilizes the autonomic nervous system that controls the blood pressure and constriction of blood vessels.

A low salt diet of 2.4 grams of sodium per day lowers blood pressure in many that have hypertension. Doctors cannot yet predict which patients with hypertension will benefit most from a low salt diet; perhaps in ten years with our expanding genetic knowledge we will be able to tell who is most sensitive to salt. The usual salt intake is 1.6 to 3 teaspoons of salt per day corresponding to 7.6 to 10 grams. Most of the salt is in prepared food, frozen dinners, canned goods, processed foods, salty snack food like potato chips, nuts and pretzels, and restaurant or fast food. Only 20 to 30% of salt in the diet is added at the table or used in food preparation at home. Blood pressure lowering medicine is more effective than diet alone in lowering blood pressure.

Blood pressure is also lowered by more potassium found in fresh fruits and vegetables, and more calcium in dairy products or calcium supplements. The best diet for hypertension is called the DASH (Dietary Approaches to Stop Hypertension) diet. This contains all the elements listed above along with menus. The studies in which patients were on the DASH diet clearly showed that a diet low in saturated fat, cholesterol, with fresh fruits and vegetables, lowers blood pressure. The diet is low in red meat and sweets, and high in whole grain products, fish, poultry and nuts. This diet has plenty of calcium, magnesium, potassium, and fiber. The web site for the DASH diet is http://dash.bwh.harvard.edu.

In summary, eat fresh fruit and vegetables, do not add salt while preparing food, and try to stay away from high calorie, and pre-processed foods.

Summary of Best Diet for Hypertension
Eat

Fruits (but not as fruit juice)

Vegetables

Fish

Poultry

Nuts without salt

Avoid

Pre-processed food

Sweets including sugary drinks

Salt

Exercise

Physical inactivity raises the risk for hypertension. Several recent studies have shown that aerobic exercise (that increases the pulses for a sustained twenty minutes or more) lowers blood pressure. It appears that African Americans may achieve more blood pressure reduction from exercise. The reduction in blood pressure is not huge but it is significant; still blood pressure medicine may be necessary. Doctors postulate that the metabolic syndrome with its high insulin levels is reversed by the daily aerobic exercise and that is how exercise lowers blood pressure.

White Coat Hypertension

No matter how friendly and disarming a person's own doctor, the blood pressure will probably rise when he walks into the room. Your husband may wonder if he really has hypertension during days of regular activity. This issue can be resolved in two ways. You can purchase a medium priced arm blood pressure cuff and learn to take blood pressures at home. We will calibrate this blood pressure cuff by comparing the reading to ours in the office to be sure it is accurate. The home blood pressures are then what we accept as the true blood pressure. An alternative is twenty-four hour ambulatory blood pressure monitoring. A blood pressure cuff is strapped on and periodically measures and records blood pressure as a person goes about his usual day, stress at work, getting a parking ticket, sleep, and awakening early to go back to work. The blood pressure monitor gives doctors a good idea of the average blood pressure in a person's daily life. Unfortunately, I have patients whose blood pressure is always high in the office, who claim to have white-coat hypertension, and who are just not taking their medicine.

Medicine That Raises Blood Pressure

Over-the-counter decongestants such as Sudafed may raise blood pressure as do prescription decongestants (usually containing a D in the name) and often combined with an anti-allergy antihistamine. Anti-inflammatory medicine for arthritis such as Motrin or Alleve and prescription arthritis medicine may elevate blood pressure. When a person must take cortisone, we anticipate a temporary rise in blood pressure.

Special Situations

African-American patients tend to have a worse form of hypertension. They often need two or more medicines to control their blood pressure, and are six times as likely to get hypertensive complications in the kidneys and eyes. Diabetic patients also are more likely to damage their kidneys when their blood pressure is not well controlled. I have good news for both groups. The new angiotensin receptor blockers (ARBs) that lower blood pressure, such as Atacand, Diovan, Cozaar, Avapro and Micardis, particularly in combination with a low dose of fluid pill are more effective than any other drugs yet. I have patients who required three different medicines, who were able to convert to one ARB pill a day with excellent blood pressure control and no side effects.

If a hypertensive patient comes in who is young and not obese, or if the blood pressure is difficult to control, we look for so-called secondary causes of hypertension. If a blood vessel to the kidney is blocked, the kidney "believes" the blood pressure is too low based on the low flow it receives, so it pumps out powerful hormones to raise blood pressure. We may look for a tumor called a pheochromocytoma that produces adrenalin, the hormone that causes the "flight or fight" reaction.

A twenty-nine-year-old male patient had an unusual case of hypertension. He was of normal weight, fit, and had no family history of hypertension. He had a blood pressure of 200/120 that had been refractory to all classes of blood pressure medicine. Something was not right! I discovered that he had been born with an Arnold Chiari malformation. In this condition, the lowest portion of the brain is located in the upper neck rather than being confined to the skull, as is normal. This put pressure on the primitive, life sustaining part of the brain (the medulla) and caused his blood pressure thermostat to grossly malfunction. These are potentially correctable causes of high blood pressure. The majority of cases are what doctors call essential hypertension, i.e., there is no unusual underlying cause.

Medicine for Lowering Blood Pressure

Twenty years ago doctors had few options for treating hypertension, and the medications we did have caused side effects. Most of my patients still think that is true today, but it is not. Due to research doctors now have numerous medicines to lower blood pressure with minimal side effects, although several adjustments may be needed to get it just right. A combination of more than one medicine may be the best option in over half the patients with hypertension. Often these combinations are available in cost-saving single pills. Several mechanisms contribute to high blood pressure and each drug by itself can correct only one of them. When only one drug is prescribed, the body often compensates by raising blood pressure to previous levels. A second blood pressure medicine blocks this compensatory response and may allow for lower doses of both medicines with fewer side effects.

One other aspect of hypertension we are only now beginning to understand is that a person's blood pressure may be a measure or symbol of multiple minute actions within the blood vessels that are more significant than the actual blood pressure itself. The dilation and constriction of blood vessels modulates blood flow to critical organs, and blood pressure medicine affects the moment-to-moment tensions and chemical reactions in the walls of these oxygen and nutrient carrying pipes.

Before going into the specific categories of medicine the doctor may prescribe, I will address the underlying fears many patients have about taking blood pressure medicine. Often they say to me, "If I start taking blood pressure medicine, then I won't be able to stop it." That is not because of any inherent property of the medicine, but because when blood pressure is too high, it stays too high unless something is done to lower it. It a person stops taking the antihypertensive drug, unless they lost weight, the body will revert to its previous level of blood pressure.

What are the facts about erectile function in men who take blood pressure pills? First, some medications are more likely to cause this side-effect than others. Earlier, I spoke about the narrowed blood vessels all over the body with prolonged high blood pressure. The inflow blood vessels that allow an erection may become narrowed after years of hypertension so that the inflow is only rapid enough when the blood pressure is too high. Patients adjust to having high blood pressure even as the insidious damage to their blood vessels goes on with each beat of the heart. When their blood pressure is lowered to normal, they get temporary erectile dysfunction until the body adjusts. My last comment on this delicate issue is this: Many men who claim blood pressure pills adversely affected their erectile function had the problem before they ever had blood pressure medicine prescribed. Due to stigma and embarrassment, it was easier to say that the blood pressure pill was causing this side-effect. Now that Viagra is readily available, doctors can separate the two problems and treat each appropriately. Diuretics and beta blockers, two types of antihypertensive medicines, are known to cause sexual dysfunction in some patients.

ACE Inhibitors

There are six basic types of blood pressure medications. Angiotensin-converting enzyme (abbreviated ACE) inhibitors work by blocking the hormone that narrows and constricts the blood vessels. ACE inhibitors are my first choice for most patients. They prevent heart attack and stroke and may prevent diabetes in those genetically predisposed with metabolic syndrome. ACE inhibitors are the blood pressure pills of choice in diabetics because they slow diabetic kidney disease. About 10% of patients develop a dry cough or a tickle in the throat as a side-effect. If this is sufficiently bothersome, doctors stop the medicine and substitute a different category of drugs. (Another option is to use over-the-counter Nasachrom and that seems to stop the cough in some.) An uncommon side-effect, one that definitely necessitates stopping ACE inhibitors and not using them again, is swelling of the lip or tongue, called angioedema. I often confide to my patients that Mike has been on an ACE inhibitor since 1985 for mild hypertension. Both his parents had hypertension so he was predisposed to get it himself. He has suffered no ill effects from the medicine and he will likely live years longer because he takes it.

Three generic ACE inhibitors are now on the market, enalapril, lisinopril and captopril. They may be cheaper than the others, which are only available by brand name. We do not yet know if some ACE inhibitors are more beneficial in preventing heart attacks and strokes than others.

Angiotensin Receptor Blockers

A second category of drugs, similar to the ACE inhibitors but more expensive, are the angiotensin-receptor inhibitors (ARBs for short) such as Atacand (candesartan), Diovan (valsartan), Cozaar (losartan), Avapro (irbesartan), and Micardis (tellmisartan). I listed them in the order of frequency I prescribe them determined by efficacy, cost, and HMO coverage. Doctors use these when a patient has a side-effect to the ACE inhibitors, but the other actions of the ACE inhibitor would most benefit him, because the effect of these two drug categories is similar. ARBs are also the preferred blood pressure medicine for diabetics and seem to work well in my African American patients. I have been impressed by the efficacy of this group of medicines in lowering blood pressure. ARBs also have the fewest side effects although some patients complain of headache, palpitations, or nausea. Because ARBs dilate the blood vessels, they may cause a low blood pressure in the hours after deep relaxation from a general anesthetic for surgery.

Calcium Channel Blockers

Calcium channel blockers, which include verapamil (generic) and all of its brand names, and diltiazem (generic) and its brand names, are also used to lower blood pressure. Plendil, Norvasc and Dynacirc SR are calcium-channel blockers available only in brand name. Potential side effects include constipation, swelling of the feet, and depression. Verapamil may slow the heartbeat. This effect can be good or bad depending on the patient's heart rhythm. What I said about salt restriction tends not to apply to people who take calcium channel blockers. These drugs are more effective with a usual amount of salt in the diet.

Beta-blockers

Beta-blockers are yet another category of blood pressure medications. They block the adrenalin effect on the heart and lower the blood pressure by causing the heart to beat more slowly and less forcefully. This medicine works particularly well for those with palpitations and anxiety. It is preferred for patients who have had a heart attack and beta-blockers help prevent migraine headaches. A potential side-effect in men is impotence, so doctors do not usually use this medicine as the first choice in midlife males. Beta-blockers cause fatigue and depression in some, and may interact with other medicines. They do not lower the blood pressure much when used alone.

Diuretics

Diuretics lower blood pressure by decreasing the salt and fluid volume in the blood vessels. I usually do not use diuretics in my midlife male patients because they can cause sexual dysfunction. However, adding a diuretic may be the only way to control blood pressure in persons who retain too much fluid. Lasix (furosemide) is a stronger diuretic but has less effect on blood pressure.

Centrally (Brain) Acting Medicines

Blood pressure lowering medicines that work directly on the brain include clonidine or methyldopa. Doctors more commonly prescribe these for older adults.

Diabetes and Hypertension

The combination of diabetes and high blood pressure is particularly damaging. People with diabetes need to have a blood pressure less than 120/80 or the damage to their kidneys, heart and eyes increases almost exponentially. It is almost more important to have a perfect blood pressure than a perfect blood sugar if you have type II (the most common type) of diabetes.

What to Expect When You First Start Blood Pressure Medicine

When a person first starts taking blood pressure pills, he may feel fatigued. That is because his body is accustomed to a high pressure, and it takes about two months to adjust. Also, once a blood pressure medicine is started or changed, it will be at least three weeks before its efficacy is known. I advise my patients not to check their blood pressure for three weeks after I adjust their medicine.

How I Helped a Husband With High Blood Pressure

Allow me to take you through my thinking and actions in the case of a forty-eight year-old executive, a non-smoker and non-drinker, who saw me for a physical examination several years ago. His blood pressure was 160/120, far too high for such a young person and he had the appearance typical of metabolic syndrome with truncal obesity, and a bloated face. I ruled out unusual causes of high blood pressure such as a blocked artery to the kidney. I advised him to lose weight and start daily aerobic exercise. I referred him to a dietician who recommended a diet high in vegetables and fruit and low in salt. I rechecked his blood pressure in four weeks. He did not follow (nor has he to this day) my prescription for diet and exercise. I started him on an ACE inhibitor, which he tolerated well and I brought him back every three weeks for a blood pressure check. The ACE inhibitor was gradually titrated to maximum dose, but his blood pressure was still high. I had to ask if he were actually taking the medicine, and he told me that he was. I next added atenolol, a highly selective beta-blocker with minimal side effects and a different, complementary mode of action relative to ACE inhibitors. I chose a beta-blocker to block his adrenalin because he was a highly stressed, reactive individual.

His blood pressure decreased to 140/100 on these two drugs but that was still too high. Not until I added a low dose of a diuretic did his blood pressure normalize. This man was at high risk for future stroke and hypertensive heart disease until his blood pressure was controlled.

What to Look for in Research on Hypertension

Doctors suspect considerable genetic variability in hypertension. Someday a person with high blood pressure will be tested for which medicine works best for him. That will save time, expense, and prevent side effects. Another area of research is the twenty-four hour timing of blood pressure surges. Specifically, the blood pressure should be lower during sound sleep. Some people have persistent blood pressure elevations during sleep and sure enough, this correlates with increased risk of heart attack and stroke. In the future, we may be recommending bedtime blood pressure lowering medicine to this subgroup to overcome this more dangerous variable of hypertension.

I will sum up my specific advice about hypertension. Your husband should have his blood pressure checked at his doctor's office every two years. If he has "white-coat" hypertension, the term used when he can just feel his blood pressure rise as he walks into his doctor's office, buy a medium-priced blood pressure cuff for the arm (not the cheapest one, and not the most expensive one with all the bells and whistles). Check the blood pressure at home once a week or once a month. Do not be consumed by home blood pressure checking. When the blood pressure is consistently higher than 130/85 he is at risk for hypertension-related complications. His doctor will probably try weight loss and diet first. If that is ineffective, and his doctor recommends blood pressure lowering medicine, I would buy the medicine, see that he takes it daily, follow up the blood pressure, and be patient as the doctor adjusts the doses and follows your husband for undesired side effects.

Blood Pressure Lowering Medicine

ACE inhibitors

Angiotensin receptor blockers

Calcium channel blockers

Beta blockers

Diuretics

Centrally acting medicines (those that act on the brain)

Cancer: What You Need to Know to Protect Your Husband

The Simple Version

If he smokes, he has a good chance of getting cancer. Try to help him quit. Otherwise, colon and prostate cancer are his biggest risk. He needs a screening colonoscopy at age 50 (done under sedation so it isn't awful at all) and a PSA blood test yearly after age 50. He needs these tests before age 50 if he has a family history of either cancer.

The Details

To most, the word cancer means prolonged, painful death. Simply defined, cancer is the loss of control of the normal growth process of cells. Some cancers are relatively benign, such as the skin cancer removed from President Reagan's nose. Others are so malignant that there is nothing that can be done about them. Doctors sometimes talk among themselves about what they would do if they had cancer of the pancreas. Most would not take chemotherapy, knowing how little it would help, and would instead make amends, settle their affairs, and maybe go to Tahiti.

How We Understand Cancer

Cells divide and create new cells normally. Oncogenes are genes that control and order this process. If an oncogene becomes defective through tiny changes over many years, it may send out a flurry of signals to make new cells and this can cause cancer, cells that multiply and spread without normal controls. Tumor-suppressor genes, on the other hand, are in charge of cell death. If they become defective or ineffective because of too many abnormal cells, you see the same problem of uncontrolled cell growth leading to cancer. It is usually not the original cancer that causes death, but the spread of these abnormally proliferating cells to other vital organs. You may think of cancer as just one disease but it is many separate diseases with different reasons for originating, growing and spreading.

A revolution in understanding, diagnosing and treating cancer is just around the corner. Instead of several cancer genes, a computer chip can now find thousands that affect a single cancer. The significance is that some cancers, previously lumped together as a single entity, such as breast cancer or prostate cancer, will be separated into those with malignant characteristics that will kill a person, and those with more benign characteristics that can safely be watched.

Cancer Statistics

New cancer cases in this country will reach a record 1.33 million in 2003 according to the American Cancer Society. Cancer deaths will rise to 556,600 lives. Some of this is because the society is aging and cancer increases with age. Lung cancer is the top killer and will kill 157,200 people this year; colorectal cancer 57,100, breast cancer 39,800, and prostate cancer 28,900. Cancer is the second leading cause of death behind cardiovascular disease. Smoking is the most preventable cause of cancer death and will be the underlying cause of death in 180,000 people this year.

What Can a Person Do To Prevent Cancer?

I wish there were more I could tell you about health habits that prevent cancer. Everyone knows that smoking causes cancer and stopping smoking is the single most important thing a person can do to protect their health. Unfortunately, researchers have been unable to show that fiber, or a diet of fresh fruits and vegetables prevents cancer. Taking supplemental folic acid may modestly help to prevent breast and colon cancer, while taking vitamin A or beta carotene supplements may contribute to lung cancer. Drinking bottled water does not appear to be safer than tap water and we know of no good way to keep modern society's pollutants and potentially cancer causing chemicals out of our systems.

Doctors have the notion that a high fat diet may aggravate the tendency toward cancer of the breast or prostate, but that has not been proven. Prostate cancer has not been prevented by more sex or less, although studies are being done to determine if vitamin E, selenium, or lycophenes found in tomatoes may help prevent it.

The most important action to take is to get the recommended cancer screening from the doctor and to keep track of the dates these were done. A man needs a digital rectal exam for prostate cancer and a prostate specific antigen test yearly from age 50 until age 75 when it becomes more controversial. Everyone needs a screening colonoscopy at age 50 and every ten years after that. A man with colon or prostate cancer in the family should talk to his doctor about when to start screening.

What are the controversies about cancer screening? The scientific method requires doctors to constantly reevaluate what they believe to be true as new studies and new scientific information becomes available. The concern about cancer screening is that it picks up small tumors that would not be problematic in a person's lifetime and does not distinguish them from tumors that will kill a person. Removing a small tumor before it spreads is still the gold standard approach to these problems. The long-term answer is genetic analysis of cancers so that doctors can accurately predict their future behavior.

Cancer is not caused by past sins. It implies no moral judgment. It is one of those things like being struck by lightning.

Colon Cancer

Symptoms
Because I am a gastroenterologist as well as an internist, I

have seen a lot of colon cancer. A classic symptom is rectal bleeding, although it surprises me sometimes how little blood we are talking about and how easily the blood could be mistaken for hemorrhoids. A change in bowel habit is a classic symptom of colon cancer. This does not mean lifelong constipation. Rather, a patient whom I saw over fifteen years ago best describes the change. She had seen on television that a progressive narrowing of the caliber of the stool may be a cancer symptom, and she had noticed that in herself. Her colonoscopy showed a cancer of the lower colon. Other symptoms are low abdominal discomfort or bloating, and rectal discomfort—the technical term for this is tenesmus, the persistent feeling that the bowels need to move. I have had patients see me because they found a lump in their abdomen that turned out to be colon cancer. What bothers me most about this disease is that it is seldom the patients who complain about their bowels through the years who get it. The patients with colon cancer that has spread beyond cure are those who have no colon symptoms.

A sixty-year-old man with mental disease and a fungus infection of his skin saw me repeatedly for one year after joining Ochsner's HMO. Because of his mental state, he never made an appointment, but would just be standing in the hall waiting for me when I walked out of the room between patients. Therefore, we never had the time set aside to review preventive medicine and only dealt with his most immediate complaints. One day he had a small amount of rectal bleeding. He was dead within three months from colon cancer.

How Colon Cancer Develops

The cause of colon cancer is progressive, genetic changes in the cells lining the colon. Bacteria or sluggishness of the bowels does not cause it. Colon cancer gets its start as a nonmalignant polyp that, if left in place, can become malignant over 20 years. Seven percent of colon cancer occurs in people under age 50. By age 65, 1-2% of the population may have colon cancer.

Diagnosis

If a primary relative, a parent, brother or sister had colon cancer, doctors recommend a full colonoscopy 20 years before the age when the relative had the cancer. To prepare for a colonoscopy, a patient drinks a jug of GoLYTELY, a chemical liquid that completely cleanses the colon, the night before the test. The next morning, he goes to the colonoscopy suite where he is given intravenous sedation. Then a nine-foot fiberoptic colonoscope with a light on the end is passed through the entire colon. This is usually a relatively comfortable procedure in that the intravenous medication sedates the patient and makes memory about what actually happened foggy. The colonoscopist removes any polyp with a wire snare, before it has a chance to become a colon cancer.

A full screening colonoscopy is now the standard of care for routine colon cancer screening in asymptomatic patients at age fifty and every ten years thereafter if the initial screen is negative for a pre-malignant polyp. Since the flexible sigmoidoscopic exam only screens the lower part of the colon, research has shown that significant colon polyps or early cancers in the rest of the colon are too often missed by this incomplete examination. Most insurance companies (and Medicare) now cover a full colonoscopy for screening.

Hemoccults are special cardboard cards that patients take home. On three different days, following a bowel movement, they put a small amount of stool from a tissue onto the cards, and drop the cards off to be chemically checked for blood. If blood is present, the person needs a colonoscopy. Hemoccults were used to screen for colon cancer and still are at times. The problem with Hemoccults is that they can miss colon cancers and are not reliable.

Genetic testing is available for familial polyposis, a condition in which one hundred percent of gene carriers develop colon cancer. If a parent has this disease, the chance is fifty percent that his or her child will have it. Genetic counseling is important before the genetic test is done because of the profound implications for the patient, on childbearing decisions and future care (total removal of the colon if familial polyposis is found.) In the future, other genetic tests should be available for colon cancer.

I will close this section on colon cancer by telling you my own story. I have observed that patients often feel fine, then are dead in a few months of colon cancer. Last summer I went to the chairman of colorectal surgery, told him I felt perfect, and that I thought I must have colon cancer. He didn't laugh at me. He said, "Kathy, I'll do a colonoscopy on you and then you will know your condition for sure and you can make your arrangements." The preparation the night before was not too bad. The day of the colonoscopy, I received intravenous sedation. I do not remember anything about the procedure, but when I woke up, Dr. Beck told me I did not have colon cancer and I have been feeling righteous ever since. If the colonoscopy is negative, it probably does not need to be repeated for ten years. By then, we will likely have genetic tests we can do simply to tell a person if they are at risk. If you are concerned about colon cancer for any reason, I urge you to have the colonscopy.

Prostate Cancer

The Dilemma of Prostate Cancer

About 30,000 men will die in the United States yearly from prostate cancer. Many more will be diagnosed with it and treated, and the majority will never know they harbor these malignant cells.

When diagnosed with prostate cancer, a man faces the

dilemma of having choices about what to do. He can "wait and watch" and if the tumor gets worse, proceed with surgery or radiation. He can wait for the tumor to spread to his bones, and then receive a hormone shot once a month, but the hormone shots often stop working after several years. He can undergo a radical prostatectomy but the surgery could result in incontinence and impotence. He can opt for radiation therapy, but neither radical surgery nor radiation to the prostate would help much if the tumor has already spread in little clumps of cells to the lymph nodes in the pelvis. What to do depends on a man's age. If he is 60, aggressive treatment of the tumor may yield over three more years of life, whereas if the man is over age 75, aggressive treatment at best will add only a few months to his expected lifespan.

Prostate cancer would occur in all men if they lived to be 150. A few cancer cells are present in up to one third of men at age 50, but they do not cause problems. The doubling time of the tumor is twelve years so it grows slowly. Half of the men over age 85 have easily identified prostate cancer if we test for it with ultrasound and biopsy. However, after the age of 85, this slow-growing cancer usually does not affect the man.

How Doctors Find Prostate Cancer

The lifetime risk of a man being diagnosed with prostate cancer is 15% and the risk he will die from it is about 3%. I do a prostate-specific antigen blood test and digital rectal exam during which I can feel the prostate tissue, on my male patients between age forty and seventy. The PSA test is controversial, because it is not yet proven that finding early stage prostate cancer changes men's lives in terms of quality or length, and the treatment may cause impotence or incontinence. The early stages of prostate cancer may be asymptomatic, or a man may experience difficulty emptying the bladder.

Prostate cancer acts more aggressively in young men. A digital rectal exam is important because not all prostate cancers raise the level of PSA in the blood. Conversely, not all prostate cancers can be detected by the examiner on rectal exam so a PSA is also drawn. The prostate specific antigen is made only by cells in the prostate so it is also a good screening test. The normal PSA is less than 4, but should be less than 2.6 in a man under age 45, and may be higher than 4.0 in normal men over age 60. If the PSA is higher than 10, the probability of prostate cancer is over 50%. A single high PSA should be repeated to confirm the abnormal result before proceeding with ultrasound and biopsy.

I found a firm spot on the left lobe of the prostate of a forty-nine-year-old male who came in for a routine physical exam. His PSA was only 3.9, theoretically within normal limits, but he did indeed have prostate cancer. If untreated, the cancer would have spread outside the capsule of the prostate and into the bone. The urologist performed a radical prostatectomy on this patient because that provided him with the best chance of cure without a recurrence several years later. My patient is cancer free today, six years later.

The velocity of PSA change may also detect prostate cancer. The PSA should not increase more than 0.75 ng/ml/year over two years or it raises the suspicion of prostate cancer. I am currently working with a fifty-six-year-old man whose PSA was 2.2 three years ago, 3.3 last year, still within normal limits, and his PSA is now 4.1. Although the actual PSA level is not that high, I am still worried that he has cancer because of the change in the numbers. I referred him to Urology for an ultrasound and biopsy. Age fifty-six is still young, and if he has a tumor, it needs aggressive treatment.

PSA is either free in the blood or bound to protein. If the free PSA is low (0-10%), the probability of prostate cancer is higher. Emerging technology will allow doctors to distinguish malignant from benign prostate cancers by analyzing the proteins in the blood bound to the PSA. This will be useful to men with an equivocal PSA between 4 and 10 and may allow a reliable diagnosis without an uncomfortable biopsy.

Treatment

Once found, prostate cancer can be treated by surgery (radical prostatectomy) or radiation therapy. The surgeon wants to be sure the cancer has not spread outside the prostate gland before subjecting the patient to radical surgery. A PET scan that picks up the unique metabolism of tumor cells may find small nests of prostate cancer in lymph nodes so that the urologist and patient will know that the cancer has spread beyond where surgery would help. Radiation therapy of prostate cancer is becoming better with each passing year. The radiation oncologist uses highly developed CAT scan imaging with sophisticated software to precisely map the prostate. The radiation therapist can then directly aim the radiation at the prostate and avoid collateral damage to tissues such as the bladder and rectum, which are contiguous with the prostate. Also, using ultrasound, the radiation oncologist can plant radioactive seeds directly into the cancer for maximum destruction of the abnormal cells, sparing the innocent cells. In the past, radiation damage to the bladder and rectum sometimes caused urinary frequency, diminished bladder capacity, and caused rectal bleeding with diarrhea. Radiation does not allow us routine sampling of the lymph nodes of the pelvis, so tumor cells that have escaped the prostate capsule may go undetected and recur in distant locations. The incidence of erectile dysfunction and incontinence is lower with radiation than with surgery, so men often opt for radiation. My practice is to consult both the urologic surgeon and radiation oncologist when a man has prostate cancer so that the patient can hear the pros and cons directly from the doctor who would do the work for him.

In the near future, a computer chip will analyze thousands of genes in a single tumor and predict accurately which are relatively indolent and can be safely left alone, and which will spread and need aggressive treatment. This gene chip will make an enormous difference to men who get prostate cancer and the doctors who diagnose and treat them.

Screening for Cancers of the Solid Organs of the Abdomen

Ultrasound or CT scan of the abdomen screens for cancer of the abdomen although this procedure is not a benefit covered by insurance in asymptomatic patients because it is probably not cost effective. However, I advocate the use of this test as a screen for asymptomatic cancer of the kidney. Kidney cancer seems to be more common along the Mississippi River, where I live. The kidneys are the filters to the body, and I suspect that toxic chemicals cause these cancerous changes. When I practiced medicine in Iowa along the Mississippi River, we saw a lot of cancer. One year, in our town of thirty thousand, the urologists removed ten kidney cancers; I diagnosed six of them. This is an unusual number for a relatively uncommon cancer. When I lived in San Antonio, these tumors were less frequent. I now live along the Mississippi and, again, and I see more kidney cancers. Because the kidneys are located far back in the abdomen, there is no sensation of a tumor until it has becomes large enough to cause pain, blood in the urine, or a mass in the hands of the examining doctor. By then, the cancer has often spread beyond the kidney, and is one of those tumors relatively refractory to radiation and chemotherapy. Most of my patients with this tumor have died when the urologist was not able to remove it completely because it had spread beyond its capsule in the kidney. I have had my husband's and my own kidneys screened by ultrasound. We did not have kidney cancer and we both felt better knowing it. The test caused no pain, no radiation, and ultrasound is noninvasive. Sometimes cost effectiveness is not the final question—peace of mind is worth a lot.

Melanoma, a Mysterious Cancer

Melanoma is a feared type of skin cancer, fortunately the least common type. It begins in the cells of the skin that manufacture pigment. About thirty percent arise from a pre-existing mole and the rest appear on formerly normal appearing skin. Risks for melanoma are these: A family history of melanoma, 3 blistering sunburns before age 20, an outdoor occupation before age 20 three summers in a row, fair complexion, blue eyes, and red or blond hair. One out of seventy-five Americans has a lifetime risk of melanoma and 25% of these tumors will occur before age 40. It is second only to breast cancer as a cause of death in women ages 30-40.

If a patient tells me that a mole has changed, I ask the dermatologist to remove it even if it does not look cancerous to me, because patients are often much more attuned to a subtle change in their bodies. If any moles look atypical (enlarging, dark, irregular in border), I also ask the dermatologist to remove it.

A superficial melanoma is an irregular, white, red or blue, or blue black spot. A nodular melanoma is a firm round mass. Acral lentiginous melanomas, commonest in older age, are dark spots on the soles, palms, between the toes, on the fingers, or on the mucous membranes. Lentigo maligna, also commoner in old age, is a larger, growing brown spot with darker specks on sun-exposed skin. Sometimes a melanoma is none of these. I had a patient twenty years ago who had a gray spot on his forearm for one week that disappeared; then swollen glands in his neck appeared and biopsy revealed melanoma. He was dead in six months. Another woman showed our team of doctors a white lump on her back. The surgeon removed an amelanotic melanoma, a white melanoma, felt to be highly lethal.

If melanoma is found when it has only spread to the

surrounding skin, it is frequently curable with surgical removal. When the cancer grows down to the underlying tissues at 3.5 mm. below the surface, or spreads to lymph nodes, the likelihood of death within five years is 70%. Chemotherapy is used for more widespread tumors but the response is variable. Men have a greater chance of death when they get melanoma.

Melanomas are a mysterious cancer. I have seen them suddenly regress, going away for no explainable reason. When this happens, it looks like a miracle. Perhaps that's what it is, or perhaps the body's immune system wins the war with the melanoma cells. Unfortunately, in many patients the melanoma is highly aggressive and often refractory to treatment.

A friend of mine is a doctor from Michigan. Fifteen years ago, he noted a strange skin lesion on his calf. It was not black. He asked the general surgeon to remove it and the pathologist who looked at it under the microscope said it was a melanoma. Further investigation showed it had already spread to his lungs and bones. Usually, this is the kiss of death. The doctor had long practiced meditation as an antidote to the sorrows and stress of medicine. One day, when he was meditating, he felt the tumor leave his body. Subsequent scans confirmed that this happened.

I am not suggesting that some of the more horrible tumors are normally cured or disappear. That has not been my experience or the experience of other doctors. However, let me leave you with this thought. Any disease that has a spontaneous remission, as in the melanoma case above, also has a cure. We just have not found it yet.

Websites that are reliable sources: The American Cancer Society (www.cancer.org), the Mayo Clinic's website (www.mayohealth.org) and the University of Pennsylvania

Cancer Center's OncoLink (www.oncolink.com) are good sources of information on all types of cancers.

Beware the "bandwagon" response to new therapies for cancer eagerly announced in preliminary stages of work. Women believed that bone marrow transplants would cure their breast cancer. Subsequent careful studies showed that this drastic treatment does not help breast cancer, but only after many women had undergone this procedure on an emotional instead of scientific basis.

A Jazz Funeral for the Chicken Voodoo Man

Cancer can be one of life's greatest challenges, helping us to grow in grace. Many people recover from this disease. Others must face the truth of their own mortality (although they often have years in which to do so). Even in the very worst cases some treatment, if not an outright cure, is often available.

There are only a few cancers that are close to hopeless, such as cancer of the pancreas. But living here in New Orleans, I have come to understand that the ending of a life well-lived can be a celebration as well as a time of sadness. When a musician or poet dies, the people here have a jazz funeral for him. The Chicken Voodoo Man died at age 62. He was a prophet in the Voodoo Temple on Rampart Street in New Orleans. He had never come to me as a doctor, and I had never gone to him for advice because I was waiting for something really important to ask him. We both missed an opportunity. But I did attend his jazz funeral.

The mourners gathered outside a small funeral home in a poor section of town. The rain was coming down and we stood under our umbrellas while the close friends and family performed his final rites inside. As his ashes were brought outside and placed in a horse-drawn carriage, driven by tuxedoed men in top hats, a glorious ray of sun broke through the clouds. We started off down the street, a New Orleans brass band playing jazz and the voodoo priestesses drumming. His admirers danced behind to the music, called "second lining" in New Orleans. The band played "When the Saints Go Marching In" and a talented dancer next to me danced that city block on his hands. As we entered the French Quarter, tourists and others joined us until the crowd swelled to several thousand in number. When we reached the small spot on Bourbon Street where the Chicken Voodoo Man spoke his prophesies on Saturday night, we all walked slowly and softly as the musicians played "Just a Closer Walk with Thee." When you have helped bury someone like this in New Orleans, you understand that death is not so terrible. It is just a part of life that will come to us all sooner or later.

FURTHER
DOWN YOUR
WORRY LIST

A Heavy Subject: His Weight

The Simple Version
The key to looking and feeling good and maintaining a person's weight is 45 minutes of daily aerobic exercise to the point of being hot and sweaty. Past a certain age, carbohydrates make us gain weight. A high lean protein diet with vegetables and edible (not drinkable) fruit is best.

The Details
Obesity is defined as a Body Mass Index (BMI) greater than 30, where BMI is weight in kilograms divided by height in meters squared. Below is a chart that gives you the healthy to obese ranges for BMI.

Ranges for BMI

20-22	Best BMI, associated with living the longest
23-25	still within the acceptable range and associated with good health
25-30	Overweight, entering the zone where there are serious health risks, such as type II diabetes, heart disease, some cancers, and stroke
30 and above	Definitely at risk for all of the diseases listed above and medically defined as obese

The web site www.weightloss-basics.com, will give the BMI if you plug in height in inches and weight in pounds. Another website useful for this purpose is the National Heart, Lung and Blood Institute web site, www.nhlbi.nih.gov.

Lean muscle mass relative to fat is a good indication of how much weight a person needs to lose and probably more accurate than the scale. You can get a body fat to lean muscle evaluation at your local gym or YMCA for as little as $15.00.

The Problem: Why People Put On Weight

Being overweight is a complex problem. Human beings come in a variety of shapes and sizes, just as their ancestors came from different temperatures, climes, and food availability. Judging or blaming overweight persons is misplaced because so much of it is genetic.

The reason so many are overweight today is the combination of a genetic predisposition to store fat with a toxic food environment. High calorie, and high carbohydrate and sugar, highly processed, and cheap fast food has caused an epidemic of obesity. A sedentary lifestyle, lack of willpower, food addictions, cravings and depression may add on pounds. Stress from our sped up society also may cause chaotic eating patterns—eating irregularly while on the run, or just grabbing something without much thought or satisfaction. The health problems caused by being overweight and the money spent on dieting costs billions of dollars per year.

Hyperinsulinemia

Insulin is triggered when a person eats carbohydrates. As we age, our insulin levels go up. The more sweets you eat, the higher the insulin levels. Insulin fills the fat cells. If the insulin level is too high, a person will gain weight and feel sluggish. The object of changing eating and exercise habits is to lower the insulin level. When people do that, they feel better, have more energy, and lose weight. Even those genetically prone with overweight parents and siblings can overcome hyperinsulinemia. It takes a literal change in metabolism with aerobic exercise and a high protein, low carbohydrate diet.

As your husband loses weight, his blood pressure and cholesterol will probably normalize. The "low fat," diet is no longer believed to lower weight or to prevent heart attacks and stroke. However, almost any diet that a person sticks with does eventually result in weight loss. A vegetarian diet lowers cholesterol the most. (Beware that foods labeled "low-fat" are generally filled with hidden sugars. Otherwise, they would taste like cardboard.) Fat in the diet may not be the villain previously believed. After eating food with some fat in it, a person feels less hungry for a longer period whereas the sugars cause more food craving.

There are many potential addictions in life. We don't accept addictions to chemicals such as alcohol or cocaine; we either shun the addicts or we offer them treatment, but we just don't put up with it. But squirreling away ice cream, chocolate and sweets is an addiction just as surely. The craving for sweets will decrease after a few days away from them. A person recovering from alcoholism must resist that first drink, so someone with an eating compulsion should not take that first donut.

Medical Consequences of Being Overweight

Ideal body weights and shapes have varied throughout history and from country to country. Renoir's nudes could never get a Hollywood screen test today. So why is this a medical issue now? The medical complications of obesity are numerous and doctors discover more about this every year. Overweight people are more likely to have type II diabetes, hypertension, high cholesterol, heart disease, sleep apnea, arthritis of the knees, and earlier death. Even a ten percent drop in body weight can improve all these conditions and prolong a good life.

Many people will never reach their idealized size, but they can be healthier by losing some of the weight. Let's take the knee for example. Mike points out to his patients that the knee bears up to five times your body weight, particularly with stair-climbing or squatting. This means that a 20-pound weight loss is, in fact, a 100-pound weight loss across the knee! Or imagine how much harder the heart has to work pumping blood to supply an extra hundred pounds of weight.

Psychology of Being Overweight and Losing Weight

People lose weight all the time. The average person has tried three to five diets over the last ten years, and maybe lost over a hundred pounds. It's *keeping off the weight* that's hard both physically and emotionally.

We have to look at the causes of being overweight and come up with strategies to confront them. Many who are overweight are also over-stressed and worn out. They do not have time for themselves because of everyone else's demands on them. A healthy diet and daily exercise should be viewed as something your husband and you have the right to do for yourself. Basic self-care also means eight hours of sleep at night, and having one hour to oneself every day. Your husband may have to say "no" to something less important than his health. Coping with extreme stress can undermine the best of intentions. So if life has just thrown your family a curve, solve that big problem first and the chance of successful weight loss will be better.

Sometimes people are too discouraged to even start because they have failed so often in the past. But those who succeed in losing weight and keeping it off are the ones who have developed a routine of good nutrition and daily exercise, have a good self-image, and combine weight loss with some other change in lifestyle, such as looking for more joy in their lives and more time for themselves.

Some Tips to Lose Weight

Pack healthy snacks for your husband so he can resist the temptation to eat high fat, sugary foods when hunger strikes. He'll feel better about himself after having had an apple, say, rather than a Mars Bar.

Healthy Snack Foods Include:

Fresh vegetables and fruits

Unsalted nuts (but not in excess, as these are high in fats)

An apple or celery with a tablespoon of almond or
peanut butter

Snacks to Avoid Are:

Power bars (most of these are so filled with sugar that you
might as well be eating a candy bar, regardless of the
"healthy" and "high energy" labeling)

Dried fruits (These are filled with sugars. Therefore, trail
mix is not necessarily a good choice.)

Pastries and candy bars

Some patients are better able to establish these new routines
by joining a structured exercise and nutrition program and
need the support of a group to make lifestyle changes. They
must overcome environmental pressures to overeat,
physiologic drives to eat, and a slowed-down metabolism
that causes them to maintain a higher than normal weight. In
the end, winning the war for permanent weight loss is always
some combination of motivation, discipline and persistence.

What Should Your Husband Eat?

We currently recommend a diet of low fat meat such as
chicken or fish, vegetables, and fresh fruit. He should not eat
carbohydrates that are quickly absorbed and cause a spike in
blood sugar but rather carbohydrates that break down more
slowly so the sugar is more even in his blood stream.

Bad Carbohydrates

Anything with sugar or honey

White bread and muffins

Bad Carbohydrates (Continued)

White potatoes

Pasta

Fruit juice and soft drinks

Better Carbohydrates

Vegetables and salads

Fresh fruit (berries are low in carbohydrates)

Whole grain bread

The Key to Maintaining a Lower Weight

Daily exercise is absolutely the key to maintaining normal weight. Not only that, I think daily aerobic exercise may be the long sought fountain of youth. With exercise, people overcome fatigue, look younger than their parents at the same age, and maintain mental and physical vitality. The three pillars of exercise are aerobic (endurance), resistance (weight lifting), and stretching so as not to become stiff or muscle bound. Notice that gardening or a leisurely stroll in the sunshine with a good friend is not one of those three pillars, although these enjoyable activities are wonderful for feeling good. Most patients I talk to believe the minor exercise they get at work or doing hobbies is enough. It is not. Nor is being a weekend warrior, one who exercises only on Saturdays and Sunday. I get up every morning at 5:30 and run on the treadmill thirty minutes, and then use the cross aerobics elliptical trainer (which is a seated-position stair stepper on a slant) for resistance training, and lift light weight for my upper extremities. If I do not feel hot and sweaty, then my mission is *not* accomplished. To have the self-discipline, exercise has to be a routine. The question, "Do I want to do this today?" is not relevant.

I "game the system" by recording programs on the VCR or viewing public television tape series. On the cross aerobics trainer I can work out the large muscles of the thighs and buttocks and read my journals or books at the same time (therefore, being heedless of "suffering" during aerobic exercise). For those who do not wish to make an investment in home equipment, join a gym or YMCA close to your home and take advantage of the many programs, classes, and machines they have to offer. Health clubs are so popular these days, I'm sure there is one not more than 10 or 15 minutes from your home.

When people do not exercise, they undergo an alarming change in body composition with aging, as can be seen by a comparison of CAT scans taken through the thighs of younger and older persons. The lean muscle diminishes to little ribbons and body fat increases dramatically. The only way to avoid muscle loss with age is to exercise five to seven days a week for preferably an hour. If your husband is so out of shape that ten minutes of walking seems daunting, then he should start with five minutes and build up. You'll be surprised how quickly he can get up to an hour.

Mike, as an orthopedic surgeon, does not recommend jogging over age 40 because of injury from the impact to the knees and spine. He also counsels avoiding high-risk competitive sports like basketball over age 40 because of the ankle and knee injuries. For aerobic fitness he suggests the treadmill, steppers, elliptical trainers, swimming and cycling. The concept of "cross-training" or simply mixing up these various aerobic activities, combined with light weight training, is a particularly sensible strategy for the midlife group.

How Your Doctor May Be Able to Help You

Medicine to Help Lose Weight

With weight loss, there's the initial struggle and then there's maintenance. Some patients may need some pharmaceutical help to get started losing their excess pounds. Appetite suppressants have gone in and out of vogue. A healthy suspicion for "diet pills" is still wise. Look no further than the heart valve problems caused by Redux and Fen-Phen. But I still prescribe appetite suppressants in some patients to get them started on a weight loss diet. Phentermine 37.5 mg, 30 mg, or 15 mg, 1 tablet each morning for 2 to 8 weeks, has been available for over 30 years, so we know its side effects. Brand names include Adipex-P, Fastin, or Ionamin and range in cost from $48.99 to $58.99 monthly. Phentermine is potentially addictive, though not as much as the old amphetamines, so it is FDA approved for three months use only. It does not damage the heart valves the way newer appetite suppressants do, although it may raise the blood pressure or cause sweating. The dieter takes a pill each morning, and feels a surge of energy that should be converted into using the treadmill. Another side-effect of phentermine is a jittery feeling. I warn my patients that if they feel angry or confrontational while taking the medicine, they should stop it.

Wellbutrin SR (buproprion), 150 mg. twice daily, is an anti-depressant that has enabled some to lose significant amounts of weight. Perhaps it lessens cravings, because it is also sold as Zyban to help smokers kick the habit.

Glucophage (metformin) is a medicine used for diabetics. Currently doctors are trying it in some patients with metabolic syndrome (tendency toward diabetes, truncal obesity, hypertension, high triglycerides and low HDL). It allows glucose to be used more efficiently and stored as fat less effectively.

I tell my patients that it is safe during those first few weeks to eat much less than they are accustomed to with an emphasis on protein foods and fresh vegetables. In the olden days, the saints prayed and fasted two times a week, and it didn't seem to hurt them. (Skipping a meal may lower the insulin levels.) I give men this list of vitamins: a multivitamin without iron, Folgard or Foltx, a combination of folic acid and vitamin B12 and B6; and carrots, spinach and kale because vitamin A is not effective in pill form and people need the vitamin A in these vegetables to preserve their vision.

Xenical blocks fat absorption, but people can spend the $100+ per month, and still gain weight by eating more carbohydrates. Lastly, over-the-counter non-prescription diet medicines are ineffective and expensive. If they contain ephedrine (such as the Metabolite diet), they may predispose a person to high blood pressure, abnormal heart rhythm, and stroke. Other herbs that have not allowed buyers to lose weight when critically studied include chromium picolinate, ma huang, chitosam, and conjugated linoleic acid.

Laparoscopic Gastric Bypass for Obesity
Increasingly, I am talking with my patients about gastric bypass surgery, since it is now available as a minimally invasive surgery through a laparoscope. A 40 y.o. man saw me last week for his annual physical exam. He had poorly controlled diabetes, took two medicines for hypertension, had sore knees, and weighed 312.5 lb. He had dieted many times. I asked him if he had thought about laparoscopic gastric bypass. He said he had already attended a seminar about it. He wondered how safe it was and what he could expect from the surgery. My overweight patients are often interested in this surgery but are shy to ask about it.

How the Gastrointestinal Tract Works
Food is swallowed into the stomach. The stomach and its acid do not digest food; the stomach only receives food and grinds it so that it passes as a liquid into the 30 foot long small intestine where the digestion takes place. Food is broken into elemental particles from carbohydrates, fats and proteins, and transported by specialized uptake systems through the intestinal lining. From there the calories and

nutrients go to the blood stream, the liver, and then are distributed in the rest of the body. After the indigestible material passes through the small intestine, it moves to the colon (also called the large intestine). Although some water is absorbed, the main purpose of the colon is to store waste, then eliminate it. Gastric bypass surgery minimizes the receiving capacity of the stomach and bypasses a significant part of the calorie and nutrient absorbing portion of the small intestine.

Who Should Consider Gastric Bypass?

Gastric bypass is for persons more than 100 pounds overweight, or who have a body mass index of more than 40. The average weight of patients undergoing this surgery is 340 pounds. These are people who have not been able to lose weight with diet and exercise, and have medical problems from obesity such as sleep apnea or hypertension or knee arthritis. The patient must meet with a psychiatrist before having surgery to be sure he can psychologically handle the big change in body image that will follow this operation. The person also has to be able to follow the instructions of the surgeon and the dietary restrictions necessitated by the surgery.

Patients who have this surgery range in age from 16 to 70 and average age 38. Insurance covers at least half the surgeries, a cost of about $15,000.

What Will the Surgeon Do?

After surgery 10% of the stomach is left to receive food and the rest is bypassed. The opening of the stomach outlet is about the size of a nickel. After surgery, a person can eat one cup of food at a time and highly refined sugars are harder to digest. Ten to 20% of patients need a second operation to improve the result of the first surgery. The nutritional supplements the doctor prescribes are important. Later, after the weight is lost, many patients opt for surgery to remove the loose hanging skin that used to be filled with fat.

The surgery is often done through minimally invasive laparoscopic surgery. The surgeon operates through a number of smaller holes with a fiberoptic scope while viewing the organs on a video to guide his movements. Because there is not a large incision, patients have less pain and difficulty healing after surgery. If there are no complications, a patient may go home in three days or less.

What to Expect from the Surgery

Patients lose 60-80% of their excess weight within the first year. About 70% normalize their blood pressure without medicine, 80% normalize their cholesterol, and up to 90% of diabetics go into remission. Asthmatics are able to breathe more easily and patients have dramatic relief from sleep apnea where the airway blocks off at night. Stress incontinence, low back pain, knee arthritis pain, and acid reflux all improve.

The surgery is designed to last about 18 months so people don't go on losing weight after they are back to normal size and the outlet of the stomach stretches to the size of a lemon. At first the bypassed part of the upper small intestine doesn't absorb food but food absorption improves over 18 months. Patients must take vitamin and mineral supplements and have periodic checkups. Patients must follow a careful diet regimen that becomes more lenient with time.

Vertical banded gastroplasty restricts the size of the stomach with a band around the upper part. I have not seen many successes with this and the band can slip into the wrong place.

What Are the Complications?

Potential problems with laparoscopic gastroplasty include nausea and vomiting, gallstones from rapid weight loss, diarrhea after rich meals, constipation due to the smaller volume of food consumed, or a blockage at the surgically changed stomach outlet. One out of 200 patients may die from the surgery.

Writing a Prescription for Weight May Have Tax Benefits

A new IRS ruling states that obesity is a disease, with or without the consequences of hypertension and heart disease. Therefore, out-of-pocket costs for some weight-loss programs are a deductible medical expense. Of course the deduction for medical expenses is far from generous. It must exceed 7.5% of the adjusted gross income. However, I am happily writing prescriptions for fitness centers and weight loss programs.

Warning: Medicines That Cause Weight Gain

Most anti-depressants can cause weight gain, through increased appetite and other mechanisms less well understood. The older anti-depressants such as amitriptylline, nortriptylline, and doxepin and a newer anti-depressant called Remeron (mirtazapine) are known to cause weight gain over time but I have patients who have also gained on the SSRI anti-depressants such as Paxil (paroxetineHCl), Zoloft (sertraline) and Prozac (fluoxetine). Celexa (citalopram) or Lexapro (escitalopram oxalate) seem to cause the least weight gain. Some psychiatrists are adding anti-psychotic medicine to anti-depressants and these medicines cause rapid weight gain. In contrast, the anti-depressant, Wellbutrin (buproprion) is sometimes used to help achieve weight loss.

Steroids (cortisone) by injection or taken orally, cause fat to accumulate in the central part of the body. The diabetic drugs, insulin, sulfonyurea drugs and thiazolidiinodiones (i.e. glypizide, glyburide, Amaryl, and Avandia) cause weight gain. In contrast, one-third of patients taking Glucophage (metformin) lose weight.

Some people are convinced they have slowed metabolism due to an underactive thyroid. If they are concerned, I order a thyroid blood test to find out for sure. If a person is taking the correct amount of thyroid replacement even though they once had an underactive thyroid, they should be able to lose weight as easily as anyone else. I do not recommend using a history of thyroid disease as an excuse for failing to lose weight. There are other more logical reasons.

The Leptin Story

In 1994 scientists found a gene in mice that coded for leptin, a protein that delivers the message to the brain from fat cells, that the body is not starving and the appetite is satisfied. A strain of mice that lacked leptin became obese, only to lose the weight again when they were given leptin. This turned out to be less simple in humans. Some obese humans have a genetic resistance to the leptin message of satiety, which is different than a simple leptin deficiency that can be supplemented.

However, the discovery of leptin was proof that there are genetic controls over how much a person weighs. In recent years scientists have identified neurologic and metabolic signals between the intestine, adipose tissues, and brain. There are signals that tell the brain the body has had enough after each individual meal and there are other signals that tell the brain when the body weight is low, normal or high.

One such signal is ghrelin, a peptide or small protein that is made in the stomach. Ghrelin levels rise just before eating, probably notifying the person that he or she is hungry. A rise in ghrelin when a person begins dieting may contribute to the hunger from dieting and lack of sustained success of most diets. A permanent decrease in ghrelin after gastric bypass surgery for obesity may be the reason people are able to lose a large amount of weight and keep it off.   Doctors are looking for a drug that would neutralize ghrelin for appetite suppression.

Presently, researchers have identified over sixty genes that regulate body weight and may be targets for weight loss medicine. In time, there will likely be more than one hundred named genes that predispose a person to weight gain.

It is well worth it to lose weight and start an exercise program at any age. Aside from stopping smoking, there is no more important step a person can take toward maintaining health and appearance. Starting is usually the hardest part, but once underway, weight loss can be a total lifestyle change. Healthy weight maintenance is a life-long commitment. Lastly, help is on the way. There are over one hundred drugs currently in development that target different aspects of the genetic characteristics that predispose a person to obesity. For example, scientists have very recently found the gene for the on-off switch that controls the size of individual fat cells. Drugs based on emerging genetic findings should be available within the next six years.

Calorie Counting
(I don't have the time to count calories personally so I put this at the end only if you are interested.)
To approximate daily calorie use, multiply the number of pounds by 12. (Our dietician does a more precise calculation called the Harris-Benedict equation. Total energy expenditure for the day = 852 + 5.7 x weight in pounds + 5.6 x height in inches - 6.1 x age in years.) Someone who ingests even slightly more calories daily than they use will store body fat. To lose weight, a person must burn more calories than he or she takes in. Our dietician takes a diet history. She finds that many people forget sugary drinks such as fruit juice when they estimate their caloric intake. (Orange juice, for example,

is 11% sugar.) She then calculates the baseline energy (calorie) needs by a person's height, age, and activity level. In her formula, to maintain weight, she multiplies the daily estimated caloric expenditure by 1.2 if sedentary and 1.3 if walking regularly. She recommends that a patient buy a calorie counter book, and take a three-day average—including a weekend day since many of us eat differently on the weekend. To lose weight, subtract 500 calories a day from the daily average calories to achieve a sustainable weight loss. A weight loss diet allows twelve hundred to fifteen hundred calories a day for women and sixteen hundred to two thousand calories for men.

Lean protein, including all fish, canned fish packed in water, skinless chicken, and lean red meats are excellent for weight loss. Complex carbohydrates such as fresh vegetables are slow to digest and do not stimulate insulin production. Twenty-five to thirty percent of a weight loss diet should consist of fat, but choose the *right* kinds of fats. Monounsaturated fats, including olive, canola, and peanut oil, are best for lowering the cholesterol. Polyunsaturated fats, such as a small amount of mayonnaise, are also not harmful. Saturated fats, including all animal fats, butter, lard, coconut and palm oil, and whole milk dairy products, are not as healthy and should be eaten in smaller amounts. Trans fatty acids used to harden margarine are probably not healthy in any but small quantities.

There are three basic food substances with different caloric density. Carbohydrates (sugar and starches) and protein (lean meat and some vegetables) have four calories per gram in contrast to fat which contains nine calories per gram. Low fat diets were popular in the previous decade. But people have to eat something because no one can survive for long on just air. So people supplemented the low fat diet with simple carbohydrates, causing higher insulin levels, and many gained weight. High protein, low carbohydrate diets are in vogue now. Along with daily aerobic exercise, the goal of the high protein low carbohydrate diet is to gradually shift the metabolism to maintain weight loss. Doctors and dieticians do not know the best combination of protein, fat and complex carbohydrates and it probably varies from person to person. Research is in progress to get scientific answers to the question, "What should I eat?"

And yes, there is something "new under the sun." Many of my patients who want to lose weight tell me their resolve weakens at suppertime when they have worked hard all day and their hunger peaks. They do not have the energy to go to the grocery store and prepare a healthy meal. An alternative for the evening meal is to stop by a Subway sandwich store. They hand out a nutritional and dietary guide and show photographs of persons who have lost substantial weight by making an evening Subway dinner   part of their weight loss routine. Subway seems to be the healthiest fast food and a quick way to satisfy hunger for the evening.

Psychology to Help You

Stress and too many demands are reasons patients cannot get on a healthy diet and daily exercise program.

Believe that you can change established behavior.

Look at this as something you are doing to be good to your husband and yourself.

Decrease stress with meditation, simplifying the life style, and saying "no" to what is unnecessary.

Nutrition Advice

More lean protein

Slowly digested carbohydrates

Some fat (unsaturated is best)

Declare yourself allergic to sweets

Avoid alcohol

The Key to Weight Loss —Exercise

Aerobic exercise 60 minutes a day 5 to 7 days a week

Resistance or weight-lifting to increase muscle mass

Stretching so as not to become stiff or muscle-bound

Diabetes

The Simple Version

If your husband has a family history of diabetes and is overweight, his doctor should check a fasting blood sugar for diabetes. He needs a high protein, low carbohydrate diet to keep his weight down and daily aerobic exercise.

The Details

I understand diabetes far differently than I did in medical school. You probably think diabetes means a high blood sugar, but that is only the tip of the iceberg. Diabetes is a lifetime of habits in a person genetically predisposed to gain weight. It starts when a child is given a donut for breakfast, French fries at dinner, and is encouraged to clean his plate or smiled at when he asks for other people's food at the table. (A healthy appetite, don't you know.) The child may be given candy to appease him or her either because the parent doesn't know better, or is too busy to attend to other emotional needs and fills the void with sweets. That child, with the plump cheeks and waist (called baby fat well into the teens) is not encouraged to run and play outside, but plunked down in front of a television to keep them out of their harried parents' way. By the time that little kid is 8, he or she has high insulin levels and insulin keeps packing more fat into the fat cells. This vicious cycle goes on twenty more years by which time the young adult is declared a diabetic. We have a lot of pills to treat diabetes, but what does that person need first? The child in whom hyperinsulinemia, or metabolic syndrome started before he ever could make an informed choice, needed a parent who was informed, who cared enough to emphasize fruit, vegetables, lean meat, and who played with him outside on sunny days.

Type II diabetes is associated with high sugar intake, little exercise, weight gain, hypertension, high triglycerides, low

HDL (good kind of cholesterol), high LDL (bad kind of cholesterol), and a propensity toward heart attack and stroke. Once the metabolism for this entire condition is in play (genetics, sugar and no exercise), the person is probably suffering the toxicity to the blood vessels and nerve cells that accompany diabetes no matter what the actual blood sugar is.

More than 100 million people in the world today have diabetes and that number will likely double in the coming decade. Diabetes comes in two flavors. Type I diabetes (too little insulin) accounts for 5-10% of cases. Type II, which is based on a different physiologic problem (high insulin levels to which the tissues have become resistant, and obesity) accounts for the rest of cases. Type II diabetes has increased almost 40% in the last ten years. Over half of new cases are individuals in their thirties, and even children are beginning to be diagnosed with this disease.

At least 5 million Americans have undiagnosed type II diabetes because they are not having symptoms and a doctor has not checked their blood sugar. The complications accumulate during the five to seven years on average it takes for a person to learn he has diabetes. Diabetics are twenty times more likely to have kidney disease, four times as likely to have a stroke or go blind, five time as likely to have a heart attack, or risk amputation of a leg later in life due to gangrene.

When a person is first diagnosed with diabetes, he or she may feel overwhelmed by the complexity of checking home blood sugars, righteously following a diet, and taking medicine or insulin on a schedule. These tasks have become easier in recent years with simpler glucometers to check home sugars, more individualized diet plans taking into account a person's lifestyle, weight, ethnicity, age, and exercise level, and more options for effective medicine to control the blood sugar.

Diabetes is medically defined by fasting blood glucose (sugar) greater than 125 mg/dl (less than 115 mg/dl is normal) and a blood sugar two hours after a meal of over 200 mg/dl. But you can look at someone and you don't need a medical degree, to tell if they are at risk for diabetes, heart attack and all the rest. Unfortunately, I see many children with the classic truncal obesity that will play out as diabetes.

Why Diabetes Matters

What is Type I Diabetes?

Type I diabetes usually starts before age 40. In type I diabetes the insulin producing cells in the pancreas are destroyed, perhaps by a virus or a person's own antibodies directed against pancreas tissue. The pancreas is an organ that lies behind the stomach and manufactures digestive enzymes as well as insulin. Type I diabetic patients must take multiple daily injections (MDI) of insulin to carefully control blood sugar as that helps to prevent the serious complications that often appear by middle age or sooner. This usually means from three to five insulin injections daily to maintain nearly normal blood sugars at all times.

The remarkable thing is that a person can be going along in life, happy as a clam at high tide, and then their pancreatic cells that produce insulin and modulate the blood sugar fail suddenly and completely. This is exactly what happened to Mike's brother Larry. I'll let Mike tell the story.

> *"My brother is two years older than I. When we were growing up he was both a very good student and a spectacular athlete. He was long and lean and boy could he jump. Larry went to college on a full-ride track scholarship and then on to grad school, also on a scholarship. This was during the Vietnam War, so he took the ROTC approach, figuring that if his number came up, at least he'd be an officer.*

"Luckily, the Asian war ground down before he got called, but he enjoyed the Army and made a career out of it. He was a computer expert but had all the usual junior officer staff jobs. When he was in his early thirties, he was stationed at Fort Campbell, Kentucky, undergoing further training. One day he was playing eighteen holes of golf; the next it was a struggle to finish nine. He thought he just had the flu or some other minor illness, so he reported to the camp dispensary. They checked him over, drew some blood and said they'd get back to him. The next day while he was taking a test, he found himself struggling to maintain his concentration. He felt as if his brain had a cloud in it, he was thirsty beyond thirst, and he had to pee every few minutes. Someone from the dispensary called with the results of his blood sugar from the day before. It was over 700 (normal less than 115)... quite elevated. They took him out of class. The next thing he remembered was waking up in the ICU at Walter Reed Army Hospital. In other words, his diabetes had presented with what we call 'diabetic coma' or 'ketoacidosis.'"

Without insulin, sugar (glucose) is unable to leave the bloodstream for storage in other tissues such as muscle or fat. Patients with type I diabetes require insulin shots because they have a deficiency of insulin. They are prone to diabetic ketoacidosis, if they miss a dose of insulin or have an infection. Since the glucose cannot enter the cells without insulin, the cells are glucose poor while the blood is glucose rich. Even if diabetics have not had a meal for hours, the liver manufactures glucose and they need a maintenance dose of insulin. Mike continues:

"This was not the last time my brother lapsed into a diabetic coma. Seven years later I got an emergency phone call from my sister-in-law. He had gotten the flu

and, over the next few days, just seemed to go downhill. He was vomiting and, as his blood sugar rose and his thinking clouded, he decided that he shouldn't take his insulin. He was worried that he might overshoot and have a hypoglycemic reaction. When his wife went upstairs to check on him, he was lying there passed out and blue. She called 911. When the EMS guys got there, Larry's blood pressure was in the low 60s, he was barely breathing and he was unresponsive. Getting down the stairs was a chore since he was about 6 foot 5 and by now weighed around 285 pounds.

"When he got to the ICU his blood sugar was the highest I've ever heard: 2016! He also had other problems. Normally, the body closely guards certain blood parameters such as its acid/base balance (or pH) and its thickness (or osmolality, we call it). Both Larry's factors were critically off the charts. For the life of me, I don't know how he survived this. His kidneys even shut down temporarily, but bounced back.

Miraculously, Larry was up and walking by the time I arrived in Virginia, but I had the feeling this wouldn't be the last of his problems. Here was a very intelligent guy who was compulsive about measuring and managing his sugars, and yet he just couldn't keep from crashing."

A person with type I diabetes must understand his disease, check his blood sugars regularly, work closely with a specialist in diabetes, and lead a more complicated life than the rest of us or problems this severe can recur.

What is Type II Diabetes?

Type II or adult-onset diabetes accounts for the other 90% of patients with this disease. In Caucasians, it usually appears after age 40 but may be seen as early as the teen-age years in African Americans, Hispanics, Native Americans and Caucasians afflicted with severe obesity. Genes predispose a person to get this type of diabetes. If your parents or siblings have type II diabetes, you can prevent it in yourself by daily aerobic exercise, keeping your weight down, and not eating sugar.

Type II diabetics usually have as much or more insulin than the average person but their tissues are resistant to it so that the glucose does not leave their bloodstream, thus their high blood sugar levels. In most cases, type II diabetics have excess body fat, especially in their abdomen. If a patient finds out that he has type II diabetes, promptly sheds the weight and exercises every day, he can often put his disease in remission without medicine or insulin shots and avoid suffering diabetic complications. Type II diabetes may manifest during pregnancy. While it needs to be treated during gestation, the mother's blood sugar will usually return to normal after delivery, but more than half of these women will eventually become diabetics. Children born to mothers with gestational diabetes are more likely to have type II diabetes later in life.

Symptoms of Type II Diabetes
The symptoms of diabetes are increased thirst, increased volume of urine, fatigue, weight loss, tingling extremities, blurred vision, difficulty healing minor cuts, or frequent infections. Gum (periodontal) disease may also signal a failing immunity due to high blood sugars. Type II diabetes is often undiagnosed for at least several years.

Because the disease runs in families, a person might suspect he has diabetes if a parent or sibling had it. A multitude of genes cause it, not just a single one that could be cut out and replaced. However, I must emphasize that type II diabetes is a lifestyle problem of too much food and not enough exercise. Our genetic make-up is the same as it was ten thousand years ago when our forebears had to be in shape to run away from tigers, catch their own meat, gather berries, and fast a few days when the hunt and gather was unsuccessful. Our genes may never adapt to driving the car to the corner McDonald's.

Complications of Diabetes

Diabetics are at high risk for heart attacks and stroke. The risk is equivalent to that of persons who have already had one heart attack or stroke, i.e., greater than 20% in the next ten years. All blood vessels can be a target for this pernicious disease. When a diabetic also smokes, has high cholesterol, and uncontrolled high blood pressure, he or she is at very high risk for heart disease.

I remember a case twenty years ago. A forty-eight year old man with diabetes, high cholesterol, high blood pressure, a two-pack-per-day cigarette habit, and a weight of 300 pounds came to the emergency room with chest pain. I admitted him to the ICU for a heart attack. Twenty years ago doctors were not yet doing immediate catheterizations to open a closed coronary blood vessel, but I treated him with as much sophistication as we had then. He improved for the first forty-eight hours, then early Sunday morning had chest pain again. I rushed to his bedside, but as I stood beside him, his heart attack progressed through the wall of his heart, his heart ruptured, and he died. I was helpless to save him.

When I met with his wife shortly thereafter, she said, almost matter-of-factly, "He knew he would die young with all the sweets he ate, his weight, and his smoking." I felt sad that I lost this patient, but I have come to understand that the doctor can only do so much for the diabetic patient. The patient must help himself. Even though following a doctor's recommendations, being faithful to meal plans, and exercising makes life more complicated, this is a diabetic's only hope for long-term survival.

Other circulatory problems include narrowing of both the large and small blood vessels in a diabetic's feet. Claudication or pain in the calf while walking may be the first symptom. A diabetic's narrowed blood vessels may cause impotence. Smoking also increases the chances of these complications, and good control of blood sugars, cholesterol and blood pressure prevent them.

Diabetics need to have a lower cholesterol and blood pressure than non-diabetics to prevent heart attack, stroke and poor blood flow to other parts of the body. The total cholesterol should be no higher than 200 mg/dl, the HDL or good kind of cholesterol should be over 40 dl/mg, and the LDL or bad kind of cholesterol should be no higher than 100 mg/dl. A diabetic should have a lipid profile (total cholesterol, triglycerides, HDL and LDL) every year. If diet and exercise alone do not achieve these levels, drugs need to be used to aggressively lower the cholesterol. Similarly, the blood pressure in a diabetic should not be higher than 120/80 as an average. Blood pressure control in diabetics is probably as important as maintaining near normal blood sugar. The blood pressure medicine categories of choice are angiotensin converting enzyme (ACE) inhibitors or their relatives, angiotensin receptor blocking (ARB) medicine. These two medicines not only reduce heart attack and stroke in diabetics, but may prevent type II diabetes in the first place in those genetically predisposed.

Nerve Damage from Diabetes

Diabetes damages the nerves, especially those at the ends of the limbs, particularly the feet. We call this condition peripheral neuropathy. Amputations and gangrene are more common in diabetics primarily because of this nerve damage and decreased blood flow to the extremities. A diabetic's decreased feeling in the feet can lead to ulcers caused by poorly fitted shoes, burns from bathing in water that is too hot, or trauma from walking barefoot. If the feet are numb, the patient may not feel the pain from an injury. This means that small injuries can become big problems.

The last stage of this damage is a Charcot foot, originally described by Dr. Charcot in the 19th century. In this condition many small fractures that have gone unnoticed by the diabetic patient can eventually destroy the foot and ankle. The poor patient simply can't feel that his foot is getting beaten up. Eventually, the foot becomes red and swollen and may masquerade as an infection. A plain xray makes the diagnosis clear, but the outcome is poor. This condition commonly leads to an amputation.

Other nerves can be damaged by diabetes. If the nerves that control the emptying of the stomach are damaged, food is absorbed erratically and the patient vomits and he has high and low blood sugars.

One of my diabetic patients was a country gentleman from the bayous of South Louisiana. I first saw him when he was 69. He had driven up with his wife through the swamps and Spanish moss because of Charcot joints from poorly controlled type II diabetes. His feet had become numb and functionless over the years.

His ankle bones and joints had been nearly destroyed. Our orthopedic foot and ankle specialist tried to save his feet instead of amputating them, even though they were so badly damaged. He also had many other complications from his disease. When I performed his pre-operative evaluation, I discovered that his mild shortness of breath with exertion was the result of blockages in all his main coronary arteries. He had to undergo quadruple bypass surgery. His kidneys wept protein and could not discharge his chemical blood waste, he often vomited because his stomach would not empty properly, and he was nearly blind from what the diabetes had done to the blood vessels in his eyes. The only part of him not ravaged by diabetes was his fine disposition.

I corrected all the problems I could and our diabetic endocrinologists worked closely with him to control his blood sugars but, to a certain extent, it was too late. We saved his feet from amputation, but he is wheelchair bound for the rest of his life. Because of him and many others like him, I feel passionately about telling you to *do something* about diabetes while you still can. Have your husband's blood sugar checked, help him keep his weight down, don't bring sweets into the home, and make it easy for him to exercise regularly. If he has a family history of diabetes, or is simply overweight and under-exercised, he could be tending toward type II diabetes.

The story of Tommy Jackson, who works with Mike at the Ochsner Clinic illustrates how even those of us who should know better sometimes require a pretty extreme wakeup call to modify health behaviors. Mike shares this story:

> *"Tommy Jackson is a 57-year-old African American orthopedic technician who has worked at the Ochsner Clinic Foundation since 1967. Just to put that in perspective, that was the year I started my senior year in high school. Tommy is from a small town in the Mississippi Delta country, and I guess you could say that his family "used to be in the cotton business." Tommy is that remarkable combination of a gentle temper in a powerfully strong body, with a work ethic that doesn't include the word "complain" or any of its synonyms. If you look up "dedicated" in the dictionary, there's a picture of Tommy Jackson. Over the last 30 years, Tommy has scrubbed with every orthopod who has worked at the Ochsner Clinic*

Foundation, so you can imagine how I felt when I stood in the clinic one morning looking at his gangrenous foot.

"Kathy had recently diagnosed Tommy's diabetes. Even though she'd gotten the diabetes under control, he still was a smoker. He'd developed what for the rest of us would have been a minor fissure between his toes. But in his case, over the span of a single weekend, it had progressed from a little sore to a raging gas gangrene that had eaten away half his foot. I knew that if I didn't cut off a good part of his foot, and pronto, there might not be a Tommy Jackson to fuss over.

"We got him to the operating room as soon as we could and I amputated the front of his foot up to about the middle of his arch—what we call a 'transmetatarsal amputation.' Because of the severity of the infection, I left the tissues open and brought him back to the operating room a couple days later to wash it out again and close it. You might think this was a highly emotionally charged scene, your own surgical team doing a mutilating operation on one of its beloved, but you know, it's harder to write about it than it was to just do it. Surgeons feel better when they are taking action—almost any action is better than not being able to act. I think there were members of our team who just couldn't be in the room when we operated on Tommy, but there were others who just couldn't be anywhere else.

"The amputation was slow to heal. We used hyperbaric oxygen therapy, submerging what was left of Tommy's foot into a high-pressure oxygen environment every day for quite some time. Eventually, we had to go back once more to the

operating room where I amputated still more of the bone that had become infected. Once I did this, he healed. He was left with not much more than an ankle and a heel, but he had something he could walk on.

"True to form, Tommy took this as a wake-up call. He stopped smoking (with Kathy's help and a little Zyban) and he started working out. We fitted him with a special shoe inlay that aided his ability to walk. He was back at work six months after this all started. That was three years ago. Today, he is still at the surgeon's side. Just as he has been every working day for the last 34 years."

Diabetes May Damage the Kidneys

Diabetes often damages the kidneys especially in combination with high blood pressure. In fact, the most common reason for dialysis or kidney transplant is diabetes. Doctors routinely screen for protein in the urine as a harbinger of diabetic kidney disease. A blood pressure-lowering group of medicines, ACE inhibitors, can protect the kidneys from diabetes, so all diabetic patients should take these unless they experience a significant side-effect.

Maintaining the blood glucose at a level close to normal is important to protect the kidneys, and herein lays my greatest angst in treating diabetic patients. A lot of times they do not do what I ask them to do. What frustrates them is that foods they once enjoyed have now become their adversaries. One spiffy, fifty year-old gentleman who came to my office periodically always had a blood sugar over 200. When I confronted him about this, he told me he had syrup on his pancakes that very morning. I carefully reiterated what he should do to keep his disease in check, then I begged him to do it. When that didn't work, I threatened him with the wrathful complications of the disease, and then sent him to a much scarier doctor than I. All to no avail. When I went to a movie a few weeks ago, he was shown on the screen before the show asking for a kidney donor because he needs a transplant.

Diabetic Eye Problems

Almost all type I diabetics and over half type II diabetics develop diabetic eye disease. High blood sugars damage the fine blood vessels at the back of the eye and they weaken, leaking blood and causing blindness is some cases. Ophthalmologists treat the abnormal blood cells by sealing them with laser. An optometrist or ophthalmologist should thoroughly examine a diabetic's eyes yearly and usually must dilate the pupil to do this.

Treatment of Diabetes

The better diabetes is controlled, the closer the blood sugar is to normal most of the time. The blood sugar should be under 120mg/dl before a meal and less than 185 to 200 mg/dl two hours after a meal. Diabetics should regularly monitor these blood sugars at home with a finger prick and a glucometer machine. Every three months the doctor will order glycolysated hemoglobin (HbA1c), a blood test that tells how well controlled the average blood sugar has been over the last three months. The HbA1c should be under seven or less. If it is within range, the whole treatment plan, diet, exercise, and medicine are working. If that number is much over seven, the doctor and patient need to go back to the drawing board and try harder to control the blood sugars.

Diet

Diabetics are "allergic to sweets". I tell patients who ask me how to lose weight to stop eating cookies, candy white bread, potatoes, white rice, and stop drinking fruit juice and Coke and other sweetened beverages. It is that simple and I spell it out.

A healthy diet is the first treatment for diabetes. I asked our dietician at Ochsner Clinic Foundation what she recommended for diabetics and she gave the standard answer. Calories should to be divided into 50-60 % complex carbohydrates (fruits, vegetables, whole grain bread), 12-20% protein, and less than 30% fat. The best diabetic diet is not so clear-cut and studies and recommendations on this are pending. For example, the old Atkin's diet (high protein, low carbohydrate), while hard to follow and stick with; drops blood sugar, weight, triglycerides, blood pressure, and insulin injection requirements. But a diabetic whose kidneys are already damaged cannot metabolize that amount of protein. A diabetic should consult with a certified, registered nutritionist yearly who has had experience setting up meal plans with diabetics. When creating any food plan to stabilize this disease, keep in mind that people respond differently to various components of diet. For example, obese diabetics are exquisitely sensitive to carbohydrates. Carbs make them fat, and thus more diabetic. Asking an already obese diabetic to eat 60% carbohydrates would be counterproductive to the goal of stabilizing the blood sugars and lowering the weight. Protein and fat have their downside also. If a diabetic has kidney disease, even in the earliest stage, protein puts a greater burden of work on the kidneys and makes the condition worse. Since people have to eat something, what about fat, much maligned as a dietary component in the last fifteen years? The downside of fat is that it is calorie dense, so may not help those who are over endowed with body weight. The upside is that it is a good energy source and allows a person's appetite to remain satisfied for longer periods. Therefore, we doctors allow more fat in the diets of those whom we counsel to eat fewer carbohydrates. The trend is to individualize the diet to the particular needs of the patient, according to his diabetic type and his body habitus. The three artificial sweeteners approved by the American Diabetic Association include NutraSweet (aspartame), Sweet One (acesulfame potassium) and saccharine.

Weight loss can be critical for managing diabetes. Even a loss of ten to twenty pounds may make an enormous difference in how easily the blood sugar is controlled.

Cutting Edge in Diabetes: What to Watch

These are unresolved issues about diabetes. The first is diet. The proportions of fats, proteins, and carbohydrates should be individualized to the patient's particular metabolism and lifestyle. The diabetic may get the same standard diet instructions that have been handed out to diabetics for twenty-five years. But a high carbohydrate diet may make diabetes worse.

Second, doctors are aggressively searching for ways to reduce complications. We are also hopeful that in some cases we may prevent diabetes altogether. Altace (ramipril), an ACE inhibitor, and a group of blood pressure lowering medicines related to ACE inhibitors called angiotensin receptor blockers (ARB's) may prevent a person from getting diabetes and definitely decreases the cardiovascular complications. Ask the doctor if your husband should be on an ACE-inhibitor, because of its role in the primary prevention of stroke and heart attack. (Cough and headache are side effects of some ACE-inhibitors. Angioedema or swelling of the lips is a rare side-effect.)

Is injecting insulin is better than ingesting three or more oral agents for diabetes? Perhaps one of the reasons that insulin is being underused now is because it is inexpensive and not promoted. An inhaled form of insulin may be available soon.

Genetic research on diabetes is progressing rapidly because it is well known that diabetes runs in families. By identifying the at-risk person early in life, the diabetic may avoid years of damage done while he is oblivious of his diabetes.

Can You Prevent Diabetes?

If a person has the genes for this disease can he or the doctor prevent that slippery slide toward obesity, high sugars, high cholesterol, and blood vessel and nerve damage? Intensive lifestyle changes, a low calorie diet, weight loss that is sustained, and daily moderate aerobic exercise prevents the onset of high blood sugars and can normalize metabolism. Also, the drug metformin (Glucophage) changes the body's abnormal metabolism that leads to insulin resistance and type II diabetes. In young people who are obviously going to get the disease because they are already overweight with a strong family history of diabetes, doctors often prescribe metformin.

The Need for Education

The key to managing diabetes has to include *educating* the diabetic to function independently with a complex, chronic disease. This requires a team approach, including the primary care physician, the endocrinologist, the diabetes educator, the nutritionist, the exercise therapist, the behaviorist, the podiatrist, the optometrist and ophthalmologist, the nephrologist, the cardiologist and perhaps more.

Normalizing blood sugar prevents complications. It is my hope that every diabetic patient can receive an education about all the aspects of his disease, what to expect, and how to deal with emergencies. Then diabetics like Larry will know what to do when they experience severe symptoms. Diabetics like Tommy Jackson will learn to be very careful of injuries to their extremities and will check their feet daily. Even though my Cajun man waited until it was too late to come for treatment, there are several people with diabetes in this family, but through education and learning about medications such as ACE inhibitors and cholesterol lowering drugs, perhaps they may avoid the neuropathy and cardiovascular disease that so ravaged his body.

For all those people out there waiting for a cure for cancer or arthritis, here's a disease for which we know the cause, how to control it and the calamities that go along with not managing it. Yet people won't lose weight, won't stop eating that Easter candy, and sometimes won't even check their feet for sores. Some say that diabetes is less a disease than a full-time occupation, and there's some real truth in that. The compensation for this full-time occupation is the possibility of living an almost normal life. In some cases, the type II diabetic can lose weight, closely monitor his sugar intake, and exercise regularly, so that he can greatly improve or even eliminate his symptoms. The key is *quick action*. If you suspect your husband has blood sugar problems, get a diagnosis and help him take responsibility for his diabetes. Don't wait until he is so sick that his body has suffered damage that cannot be repaired. The quicker you and he act, the more hope there is.

Website for Information on Diabetes
American Diabetes Association National Service Center
http://diabetes.org

Types of Pills for Diabetes
(Only of Interest to Those With Diabetic Husbands or Who Have Diabetes Themselves)
This next section contains detailed information about types of medications used to treat diabetes. If you are only reading this chapter because you think that you or a loved one *might* have diabetes and you want to learn more about it and its symptoms, then you may wish to skip this section for now. Often more than one medicine is used in combination with another oral medicine or with insulin.

Sulfonyureas
Type II diabetes is more often treated with oral medicine than with insulin shots. The oldest group of medicines is sulfonyureas. This includes Amaryl (glimepiride), Glucotrol

(glypizide), and Diabeta, Glynase Pretab and Micronase (glyburide). These drugs stimulate the pancreas to produce more insulin. The sustained-release form of glypizide lowers blood sugar with less risk of causing low blood sugar than the short-acting and less expensive counterpart. Its effect is supposed to last for twenty-four hours but may wear off sooner. For this reason, some patients need the Glucotrol XL twice daily. Glimepiride (Amaryl) has the advantage of acting for a full twenty-four hours, so it can be taken once a day. A side-effect of all these medicines is weight gain, which is counter-productive in a type II diabetic.

Biguanides (metformin, brand name Glucophage) (often the best oral drug)

Glucophage (metformin) is the first choice in an overweight diabetic because it can help the patient shed some of the weight. Metformin increases the muscle tissue's sensitivity to insulin, decreases the manufacture of glucose by the liver during the fasting state, and does not cause hypoglycemia or weight gain. Thirty percent of patients have side effects, most commonly diarrhea or bloating. About 30 % of patients spontaneously lose weight with this medicine. Glucophage treatment begins at 500 mg taken twice daily, but can be adjusted up to 1000 mg. twice daily. Glucophage XR 500 mg. is available as an extended-release form. Glucophage should not be used in patients with poor kidney, heart, or liver function or in alcoholics, and must be stopped around the time of surgery or radiology procedures using dye. It may be used along with sulfonyureas or insulin. Glucovance is a combination or glyburide and metformin. The advantage is achieving the same lowering of blood sugar with fewer total pills. Watch for other combination medicines like this.

Thiazolidinediones

Another group of drugs makes the tissues more sensitive to insulin, so that glucose does not build up in the bloodstream and is taken up by the muscle as it ought to be. These drugs may also decrease inflammation in the blood vessels that are so often the target of diabetic damage. Some patients who were taking insulin injections were able to stop their insulin as these drugs helped normalize their blood sugars. These medicines may be added as a third drug when the patient is already taking a sulfonyurea and metformin.

The first drug released, Rezulin, was taken off the market due to severe liver toxicity in a few patients. The liver damage was probably specific to the chemistry of that drug. Avandia (rosiglitazone) and Actos (pioglitazone) are chemically similar to Rezulin and patients taking them must still be checked for liver toxicity every two months for the first year. Avandia or Actos can be added as a third drug when the sulfonyurea and Glucophage (metformin) alone are not controlling the blood sugars. There are some side effects to consider, however. These medications may cause weight gain and are not recommended for patients with congestive heart failure or liver disease.

Who Needs Insulin Injections?

All type I diabetics need insulin or they will die in diabetic coma. Many type II diabetics eventually need insulin injections to control their blood sugars. Insulin is also useful for some patients who have to take a large number of pills for other conditions. For example, one patient I care for is on four drugs for his diabetes and a dozen drugs for his heart transplant, so for him, insulin is a simple and elegant solution. Unfortunately, even high doses of insulin may not adequately lower the blood sugar or prevent complications in very obese patients. Insulin injections can cause weight gain, which is at the core of type II diabetes.

Even if a person were to eat no sugar or carbohydrates, the liver manufactures too much sugar in diabetics. The liver does this at night when the innocent diabetic is sleeping and not even eating. The technical term for this is gluconeogenesis.

When doctors think of converting the patient to insulin injections, this nighttime gluconeogenesis is a prime consideration. The patient will often take ten units of insulin at night to signal the liver to stop making the sugar. The result is that his morning glucose will be normal, although he may still need one of the above-mentioned oral medicines during the day to control his blood sugars after eating.

If oral medicines fail or the regimen seems too complicated and expensive to the patient, a type II diabetic may simply be given a twice-daily insulin routine. The morning and evening doses are usually a combination of the long and short-acting insulin to level out the blood sugar. The patient, his doctor, and diabetes nurse educators can work with his blood sugars and insulin doses to perfect his personalized regimen.

Short acting insulin comes in the form of regular insulin or Humalog. The advantage of Humalog is that it acts immediately to lower the blood sugar. Patients who use regular (R) insulin as their short-acting form must take it half an hour before a meal but they often do not have the patience or leisure time to do this. So they take it right before a meal. When this happens, their blood sugar spikes high during eating and then crashes back down after the meal. Since Humalog acts immediately, it may be taken with the meal to prevent blood sugar spiking during eating.

The two long-acting insulins that simulate the baseline output of the pancreas are Humulin N that acts over 8 to 10 hours and a new 24-hour acting insulin, Lantus (glargine). Long and short acting insulin are often used together so the blood sugar is normalized during and between meals.

Insulin comes premixed as either 70/30 N/R or 75/25 N/Humalog. The patients who receive premixed insulin are those who cannot mix their own short- and long-acting insulin due to age or failing eyesight.

Insulin must be taken as a shot because it is a protein that would otherwise be broken down by digestion if taken by mouth. Insulin is easier than ever for people to give themselves. There are insulin pens where all you have to do is press a button and a pre-measured amount of insulin is automatically dispensed.

Erectile Dysfunction, Viagra, Andropause and the Hormones of Aging

The Simple Version

Viagra doesn't harm men and is probably good for them. Men do not become dependent on it and it does not stop working over time.

The Details

Men by age 40 often experience a subtle change in the quality of erections. At age 18, a man worries whether he will find a sexual partner. At age 40, he worries whether he will get a timely erection in an appropriate sexual situation, and whether that erection will be sustained.

The Mechanics of Erectile Dysfunction

The "plumbing" of erections is inflow and outflow. First, blood has to flow in fast enough through the arteries (inflow vessels) for an erection to occur. Then the veins have to clamp down at the base of the penis for the erection to be sustained. Problems getting erections occur when the fine arteries that feed the penis become narrowed. The two commonest causes of this narrowing are high blood pressure and smoking. When the blood vessels narrow, the blood flow to the penis is slower and so the erection takes longer to achieve and may be less firm. Smoking constricts all blood vessels in the body, causing heart attacks, strokes, peripheral vascular disease of the feet and (they should put this in the Surgeon General's warning) impotence.

On the other side of the plumbing equation is venous outflow. It is common for men over age 40 to have a varicocele (dilated veins) at the base of the penis. If venous outflow is too fast, the man loses his erection.

Nerve damage is another common physical cause of erectile dysfunction. Diabetics are especially susceptible to this because diabetes damages the body's nerves. The nerves that control erections run through the perineum, the part of the body behind the testicles. Long distance bicycle riders may injure these nerves with prolonged pressure. They may experience numbness and erectile dysfunction. Special bicycle seats are manufactured to decrease the pressure on this part of the body.

Low Testosterone

When men experience difficulty getting and sustaining an erection, they often wonder if they have enough testosterone or if their male hormones are giving out, just as a woman's ovaries fail during menopause. Men's testosterone levels do gradually decline from age eighteen on. Called andropause if it becomes symptomatic, this drop in testosterone does not happen as surely to men as the loss of estrogen during menopause, nor does it always cause symptoms.

The symptoms of andropause are irritability, low energy, erectile dysfunction, fatigue, decreased libido, and muscle weakness. Men will also have "menopausal" symptoms, including hot flashes and fatigue. They may experience a greater percentage of body fat relative to lean muscle, decreased concentration and memory, and even osteoporosis, just like a woman after menopause. Mild anemia is another tip off that testosterone is low. Men usually have a higher blood count than women, but their blood count "feminizes" at a lower level if they have lowered testosterone.

A *low testosterone* is classified as:
primary, meaning the testicular tissue stopped producing the hormone
secondary, meaning the pituitary gland in the brain stopped signaling the testes to make testosterone

tertiary, meaning the brain center, the hypothalamus, that controls all glands, has shut down the testosterone production.

Most cases of low testosterone are due to age. Instead of a phasing out of the reproductive cycle like ovarian failure in women, low testosterone is more likely due to lower brain signals to the testes to produce hormone (the secondary and tertiary causes).

Causes of Primary Low Testosterone Are:

Testicular disease from infections contracted years ago, such as mumps

Previous trauma to the testes

Genetic problems

Hemochromatosis (a disease caused by excess iron absorption that affects at least one out of a thousand Caucasians)

Excess alcohol use which feminizes men by creating more estrogen relative to testosterone in their bodies

Sleep apnea, which causes low testosterone, erectile dysfunction, and low libido, possibly because of lower brain oxygenation at night.

Blood Tests for Low Testosterone

Doctors can check for low testosterone with a blood test, and often order this test when a man complains of erectile dysfunction. The total testosterone should be done at least twice because it may not be accurate with just one reading. The blood level should be drawn first thing in the morning in a fasting state. If the total testosterone is less than 300 ng/dl on two occasions, it is likely that the man has a deficiency. The free testosterone test tends not to be accurate, so total testosterone is the preferred test.

When I was in the Air Force, I had a hardy, trim General

Officer for a patient. This was in the days before Viagra was available; thus I did not ask about erectile dysfunction because so little effective and satisfactory treatment was available. When I noted that his hemoglobin (blood count) was two points lower than normal, I evaluated him for blood loss, e.g. from a silent colon cancer, and for a vitamin deficiency. When I checked his testosterone, it was quite low. I treated this with testosterone shots every two weeks, since those were the days before testosterone patches were available, and his blood count returned to normal. He also reported to me that he was experiencing greater sexual vigor.

Weight Gain Can Lower Testosterone

A more common, less known cause of lowered testosterone efficacy will not be apparent from a blood test. When men acquire even ten or twenty extra pounds around the waist, that metabolically active fat in the abdomen converts some testosterone to the female hormone, estrogen. I explain this to my male patients who have noticed a decrease in erectile function and need to lose weight. It seems that nothing motivates them quite as quickly to lose the extra pounds than the thought of becoming less potent.

A fifty-year-old Air Force officer saw me for his retirement physical. Even though the Air Force demands that active duty personnel maintain weight standards or be involuntarily separated from the service, this man had let his weight increase as he anticipated retirement and less strict rules. He was concerned about the erectile dysfunction he'd experienced for the past six months, but did not put the two phenomena together. After I explained the connection, he lost that weight faster than if he had been threatened with demotion to Airman Basic (the entry level in the Air Force.) When I saw him later, slimmed down and looking ten years younger, I asked him if his other problem had improved. He smiled and said to me, "If all your treatments work this well, your patients will be truly grateful."

Physical Causes of Erectile Dysfunction

Slow arterial inflow

Rapid venous outflow (e.g. due to a varicocele)

Nerve damage

Low testosterone

Truncal obesity

Symptoms of Low Testosterone

Depression and mood swings

Erectile dysfunction

Low libido

Hot flashes

Muscle weakness

Psychological Aspects

Men do not tolerate erectile dysfunction very well. When they are less potent, they tend to worry more about themselves and life crises may begin. They become afraid that their long-term wife or lover may no longer be attractive. Or they worry that they are getting old and no longer have the vigor of a young man. These tend not to be just passing thoughts, and I take them seriously in my patients.

I bring up the issue of erectile dysfunction when doing a complete history and physical on most male patient past age 40, but usually in a roundabout and non-threatening way. When I am taking their history, and I get to questions about urinary symptoms, I simply ask them if they think they need Viagra. Usually, they will say, "No, I don't need that." Commonly they call me two days later with the telephone number of their drugstore, asking for a prescription.

Treatment With Viagra

Viagra (sulendifil) is an excellent drug. A person takes either

25, 50, or 100 mg. one hour before sex and the inflow and outflow of blood to the penis are restored to normal. My patients have been very pleased with the results. A younger man may need only 25 mg, but the manufacturer charges the same amount for a 25 mg, 50 mg, and 100 mg pill, between $8 and $9, which insurance companies do not cover. Using a pill cutter, (cost $4.50), an individual can get maximum benefit for a lower price. Don't expect free samples. The drug company does not like to give any away free because, as they explained to me, it is "like the bank giving out money."

Men worry that they could become addicted to Viagra, that it could inhibit their natural virility. This is not true. If they use Viagra a few times and the arteries, the inflow blood vessels, become dilated, men often do not need to use the medicine again for several weeks. Viagra does not lose its efficacy with time. Also, it does not cause heart attacks. Although sexual activity sometimes causes heart attacks, Viagra is not dangerous to the heart. However, men who take a heart medicine called nitroglycerin or long acting nitrates like Imdur absolutely may not use this medicine because the combination causes dangerously low blood pressure.

I have watched the medical literature and spoken to my urology colleagues about Viagra. Given the large amount of the drug being used in this country, very few side effects have been reported. Some men get a headache from dilated blood vessels and some describe a blue haze about their vision that lasts until the medicine is metabolized and released from their system.

My patients sometimes ask me the following question: If a man is depressed, because of, or in addition to, erectile dysfunction, should he take both Viagra and his anti-depressant medicine, which may have the side-effect of delaying orgasm? To my knowledge, there is no harm in doing so. One of my partners, a Ph.D. in Pharmacy, has researched this in all the pharmacology literature and there are no reports of a bad reaction if the two are taken together. Another colleague, who is a psychiatrist, says that Viagra is often prescribed to overcome the sexual side effects of anti-depressants. The alternative is to use the anti-depressant, Wellbutrin (buproprion) which does not have sexual side effects.

Testosterone Replacement

Testosterone replacement can restore energy, libido, sexual characteristics and normal function, and prevent osteoporosis in those with low testosterone. It increases muscle mass and decreases fat.

There are some possible side effects including sleep apnea, an increase in the red blood cell count that can thicken the blood and decrease flow to the brain, acne, or skin irritation if testosterone is applied topically as a patch or gel. The breast tissue may enlarge and the testicles usually become smaller. One of the biggest concerns is that a small, latent prostate cancer, common in men over age 40, will grow more rapidly when stimulated by testosterone supplements. Therefore, a PSA and prostate exam should be done before and every three months after replacement therapy is started, and then once each year. (On the other hand, the requirement to search for prostate cancer imposed by supplementing testosterone may require treatment for abnormal cells that would never have caused him any trouble in his life time.) Another problem is that the prostate may grow larger with these supplements, manifesting as difficulty urinating.

Side Effects of Testosterone Supplements

Sleep apnea

Increase in red blood cell count resulting in sluggish blood flow (e.g. to the brain)

Side Effects of Testosterone Supplements (Continued)

Growth of latent, asymptomatic prostate cancer

Prostate enlargement with partial obstruction to the outlet of the bladder and urine flow

Acne

Breast enlargement and smaller testicles

Testosterone replacement comes in three forms, 200 mg. injections every two weeks, Androderm patches applied daily, or testosterone gel. Since the injections cause a sharp peak in testosterone, 'testosterone rage' has been described, but this probably only happens in those whose underlying personality predisposes them to rage. The total testosterone level should be checked just before the next injection to be sure the dose is adequate in amount and frequency. Most health plans will cover this form of hormone replacement because it is inexpensive. The injections can be painful because they must go deep into the muscle to be absorbed.

Transdermal testosterone patches are applied to the scrotum daily after bathing because the hormone is absorbed through the skin of this area much more easily than through skin in other locations. The patches may be applied elsewhere but then the hormone is less well absorbed. These patches have the advantage of mimicking the natural diurnal variation in testosterone levels. A patient has to be motivated to apply the patches daily and sometimes they tend to fall off. Testosterone gel is more expensive but works similarly to the patch except it is more poorly absorbed so higher doses must be used. Oral testosterone in men is not presently an option. Whereas tiny doses in women are not harmful, the doses in men may lower their HDL, the good kind of cholesterol, and cause liver toxicity, and rarely liver cancer.

DHEA, a hormone that is converted to testosterone, decreases with age. It is readily available as a supplement in health food stores. The problem is the impurities. A lot of DHEA is made in Mexico and the contents are uncertain. So far, there seem to be no major side effects in men.

Growth Hormone

Growth hormone, a very costly injectable hormone, is being touted by entrepreneurial clinics as the fountain of youth. The only study looking at growth hormone in normal aging adults was printed in the *New England Journal of Medicine* over 13 years ago, looked at 12 older men injected with human growth hormone for six months, and these shots increased their muscle and bone mass slightly. The increase was so small that the researchers concluded something other than growth hormone caused muscle to turn into fat later in life. A whole industry has grown up around this study and one has to wonder about this, given the small numbers and essentially negative conclusion of this old study.

Erectile dysfunction is something men should discuss with their doctors because it is readily treatable with Viagra or may signal a deficiency of testosterone. The doctor needs first to go through a checklist of other problems (obesity, smoking, alcoholism, sleep apnea, diabetes and hypothyroidism). These days, erectile dysfunction is not the embarrassing, rare, or depressing condition it used to be. Just as the invention of eye glasses contributed to a productive life after youth, so have the scientific discoveries allowing ongoing normal male sexual function contributed to men's and couples' well-being and happiness.

Urologic Problems in Men

The Simple Version

As a man ages, his prostate enlarges and it is harder for him to empty his bladder. Burning with urination often means prostatitis. Painful blood in the urine is often a kidney stone and painless blood in the urine may be bladder or kidney cancer.

The Details

A fifty-year-old man takes his wife to a movie at the Cineplex. He buys a big gulp coke and some popcorn, finds a suitable seat and settles in for the film. But about 90 minutes into the two hour film, he realizes he's got to go. He toughs it out, because after all, it's women that have to stop every hour on a long car trip, right? The film gets over and he's down the stairs and glad when his wife says, she wants to stop in the ladies' room. He walks into the men's john and though there's a smaller line and it's moving faster, it isn't exactly moving as fast as he'd like. Then when he gets to the urinal and unzips, he finds himself standing there for what seems like an eon before he finally starts to empty his bladder. The teenagers on either side change ranks at least three times while he's emptying his bladder. And then what's this? Is it over or isn't it? He dribbles the last few drops, a pitiful finale to what used to be something he took for granted.

Benign Prostatic Enlargement (BPH)

As men pass age 40 they experience a gradual enlargement of the prostate, a walnut-sized gland that sits at the base of the bladder. The prostate's purpose is to make secretions that lubricate sperm. When the gland enlarges it can partially block the flow of urine. A man might notice a slowing of the stream of urine, a delay for a few moments before urination occurs, and nocturia, getting up at night to go to the bathroom. These symptoms are not dangerous and do not require urologic intervention. It is safe just to live with them.

If the symptoms interfere with sleep, Flomax .4 mg. (tamsulosin HCl) at bedtime relaxes the muscle at the outlet to allow complete emptying of the bladder. The herbal supplement saw palmetto varies so much in active ingredients that it is hard to say if it is of any benefit.

Most men from age 40 on, have what is technically termed post-void dribble. That means that once they have completed urination and the sphincter at the outlet of the bladder has closed, a few additional drops of urine are released from the urethra. As a man ages, the urethra begins to curve more into the prostate bed beyond the sphincter of the bladder and this acts as a second reservoir of urine. Mechanical treatment for this problem is straightforward and easy. If a man presses on the perineal body, the smooth spot behind the testicles, after urination, the urethra will then empty completely.

Prostatitis

Prostatitis is a common urologic problem. Prostatitis is different from benign enlargement of the prostate. Symptoms are urinary frequency, urgency and pain in the area of the prostate. If the prostatitis is caused by an acute bacterial infection, a man may become ill and feverish. Doctors treat the patient with antibiotics to stop the bacteria from multiplying. Since a man's primary care doctor can prescribe those antibiotics, he does not have to see a urologist for the initial attack.

Chronic prostatitis can be a more difficult problem, both understanding the cause and treating the symptoms. Bacteria may cluster around tiny stones in the prostate, causing a low-grade, chronic infection without high fever but with the symptoms of urinary frequency and discomfort. Eradicating the bacteria in chronic prostatitis usually takes one to two months of daily antibiotics, and sometimes a few additional months of suppressive doses. The term, suppressive dose, means a lower dose or frequency of antibiotics to discourage the few remaining bacteria from replicating and starting the infection all over again.

Chronic prostatitis, or its symptoms, can also be due to non-bacterial causes. For example, physical trauma may cause prostatitis. One fifty-year old male patient of mine complained of chronic perineal pain that did not respond to antibiotic therapy. I referred him to a urologist who noted that he rode a bicycle one hour every day for aerobic exercise. The urologist advised cross training, such as swimming, and that relieved my patient's symptoms.

Another patient had two highly stressful and responsible jobs that left him awake at night, worrying. He developed spasms of the muscle at the outlet of the bladder and mild secondary urinary retention. This caused his prostate to be chronically infected. The same urologist treated my patient with two months of antibiotics, and also prescribed a muscle relaxant at night to help him sleep and relax his sphincter muscle so the bladder could empty completely.

Sometimes, a patient has chronic pain in the area of the prostate and a definite cause is never found. If antibiotics improve this condition, doctors generally presume that a low-grade bacterial infection was present. If antibiotics do not improve it, then we use anti-inflammatory medicines such as Advil or Motrin.

All men experience gradual enlargement of the prostate as they pass into midlife. The official medical term for this condition is benign prostatic hypertrophy, a normal consequence of the effect of testosterone on the prostate gland. Prostate enlargement and prostatitis are not cancer, and do not become cancer. However, prostate cancer is also a common occurrence in men as they age. Prostatitis can be a vexing problem for the patient and his doctor, but in many cases, doctors are able to treat it and get relief of the symptoms of pain and frequency.

Kidney Stones

The commonest rejoinder by women when kidney stones are mentioned is, "My husband had a kidney stone!" Well, my husband also had a kidney stone. We lived in San Antonio, Texas, where the temperature often rose over 100 degrees in the summer. He was doing fifty-mile bicycle rides with younger men. Because of the dry heat, he evaporated a lot of sweat and didn't know it, concentrating the urine. I was trying to feed him healthy food so he was getting spinach every night, which is high in oxalate, a component of stones. South Texas has delicious grapefruits, so after a long ride he made grapefruit juice and drank it to rehydrate. Grapefruit is also high in oxalate.

One day, while attending a conference, he had a terrible pain in his right side and almost fainted. These episodic pains persisted, but gradually moved down into the right flank, and then the right groin. He stoically said nothing until one morning he awakened with what he described as "an elephant standing on my right testicle." He saw his doctor later that morning and was diagnosed with a kidney stone, stuck in the ureter (tube between the kidney and bladder) right where it joins the bladder. The diagnosis was easy. There was blood in the urine and a small calcified stone seen on a plain xray of the abdomen. He also had a kidney xray, known to the trade as IVP (for intravenous pyleogram), to determine how seriously blocked his ureter was. The stone was not completely obstructing Mike's ureter so his urologist gave him a chance to pass it on his own. Mike drank gallons of fluid, but the pain persisted. Finally, his urologist had to mechanically pull out the stone by passing a little basket through the cystoscope, a small fiberoptic tube with a light on the end. I saw the offending stone. It looked like a burr, and I can see why it had lodged in that tender part of Mike's anatomy. He was so relieved after the stone was out that he went two-step dancing at the Yellow Rose that night. Although two-thirds of stone victims have a recurrence, I stopped feeding Mike spinach and grapefruit, and he gave up those long rides in the hot Texas sun. He has not suffered another stone.

Foods Containing Oxalate

Spinach

Grapefruit Juice

Beets

Chocolate

Coffee

Cola

Nuts

Rhubarb

Strawberries

Tea

Wheat bran

Diagnosis of Kidney Stones

A stone passage is a remarkable event, causing pain, radiating to the groin or testicle, and blood in the urine. While the blood may just look like dark urine, the pain is often equated to labor during childbirth. In contrast, painless blood in the urine may signify bladder or kidney cancer. Men are two or three times as likely to have stones as women. Stones tend to announce themselves in the fourth decade of life. Around one-fourth of stone-formers have a family history of kidney stones.

The urinalysis most commonly shows blood cells. However, if the kidney stone is completely obstructing the ureter, the blood cells may be absent. Pus or white blood cells in the urine mean a serious problem, since an infection trapped above an obstruction in the ureter might not respond to antibiotics and can spread into the blood stream.

The patient is usually quick to identify that he has a medical problem, so many kidney stone patients get themselves to the emergency room. In addition to the urinalysis, the emergency room doctor is likely to do a spiral CAT scan, a ten-minute procedure without dye that usually identifies the offending stone. The spiral CAT scan cannot always visualize the lowest part of the ureter where it connects to the bladder. Urologists still do the IVP (kidney xray with dye) that tells how severely blocked the ureter is. (If no dye passes, it is blocked completely). If a patient has a known allergy to dye or iodine, he receives medicines to block the allergic response or takes an alternative test.

Treatment of Kidney Stones

The mechanical treatment of a stone depends on its location in the ureter and the extent to which it is obstructing it. If the stone is in the body of the kidney, it does not have clinical significance and does not require mechanical removal except in rare cases where the stone is very large. If the stone is less than 5 mm, the patient may be able to flush it out by drinking enough water to produce two liters (one-half gallon) of urine daily. Lemon juice helps dissolve the stone because it contains factors that inhibit stone formation. The doctor will send a strainer home with the patient so the stone can be retrieved for analysis if it does pass. The chemical makeup of the stone determines the strategy for preventing more.

If the stone is securely lodged in the ureter and does not pass with water and time, the urologist must remove it. The urologist may first pass a stent into the ureter to bypass the stone and allow urine to drain if the ureter is dilated (filled with non-draining urine), if the patient is in a lot of pain, or if the urine is infected. The upper ureter is above the iliac crest (known to most as the hip bone). If the stone is lodged there, lithotripsy, (shock wave therapy) is done under anesthesia to break up the stone and allow it to pass. If the stone is stuck in the lower ureter below the hip bone, the urologist may send a basket up to grasp it or use laser to destroy the stone through the cystoscope.

Recurrent Stones

As you might imagine, patients could easily tire of this ordeal if it happened more than once. Here is where the chemistry of kidney stones comes into play. Although fifty types of stones exist, the majority contain calcium salts. The lab can identify the offending materials—usually calcium, oxalate, and/or uric acid—in the actual stone. The lab can also tell from a 24-hour urine specimen what mineral a person is excreting in excess. It is not only excess minerals that cause the stones, but the lack of natural inhibitors that prevent stones from crystallizing. If a person passes one calcium oxalate stone (the commonest kind) his treatment will be to drink enough water so that he passes two liters of urine daily. The thinking up until recently was that he should also avoid calcium supplements, excess milk, and oxalate-containing foods such as spinach, grapefruit, chocolate, and instant ice tea. However, it now looks like a low salt diet is more important in preventing kidney stone recurrence.

If a person excretes too much calcium, his doctor may prescribe hydrochlorothiazide, a diuretic that reduces calcium in urine, or Urocit K, a pill taken several time a day to increase the stone inhibitors in the urine. He may be checked for hyperparathyroidism, a condition in which the calcium-regulating gland in the neck is malfunctioning. If the patient is excreting an excess of uric acid, the culprit in gout and some kidney stones, he should take zyloprim daily, a pill that blocks the formation of uric acid in the body fluids.

A kidney stone is a dramatic, painful, and memorable event. Keeping the urine dilute with adequate water intake can prevent a stone. If a stone passes into the ureter, treatment will depend on its size, location, the havoc it is causing, and whether it manages to pass on its own. If kidney stones are a recurring problem, their chemistry can be analyzed and they can be prevented with medicine.

Sleep Disorders

The Simple Version

If your husband has loud snoring and startles awake, he may have sleep apnea. This means he is not getting restful sleep, nor enough oxygen to his brain and heart.

The Details

A wife explained to me, "I'm used to the snoring. I've heard it as long as I can remember and it's rather comforting. But when he stops breathing, I just lie there awake waiting for the next breath. I think he has sleep apnea but he won't go to the doctor. And he just can't keep his legs still. They keep jumping around and he can't control it. I've tried massaging his legs, but it seems that he is never comfortable when he sleeps."

Normal Sleep

Normal sleep has two states, non-rapid eye movement and rapid eye movement sleep (NREM and REM). NREM accounts for 85% of the night's sleep, beginning with drowsiness and progressing to the deep layers of sleep. REM sleep accounts for the other 15% of sleep and is the time when a person dreams but muscle action is inhibited. REM may allow memory to consolidate. When you think about it, sleep must represent very complicated brain wiring. How else would birds sleep while they are flying over the Gulf of Mexico? It is said that dolphins sleep with half their brain while maintaining wakefulness with the other half so they can continue breathing fresh air while in the water.

How Doctors Think about Sleep Problems

People may not get enough sleep or the sleep they do get is not restful and normal. Sleep problems include difficulty falling asleep (sleep onset insomnia), staying asleep (sleep maintenance insomnia), or daytime sleepiness even after what seems to be an adequate night's sleep. When a patient is observed by video in a sleep lab, the reasons for these problems may be myriad.

Commonly Americans do not get enough sleep. They develop a sleep deficit over the week and recover the sleep debt over the weekend. A nap during the day only restores the sleep debt that accumulates after a few hours of being awake. On average, people need one hour of sleep for every two hours of wakefulness.

One third of the U.S. population complains of insomnia and one-half of insomniacs consider it a serious problem. In addition to poor concentration and decreased memory, insomnia causes irritability, decreased enjoyment of life, a lessened sense of well-being, and difficulty coping. Without enough sleep, people are accident prone. With age, the length of drowsiness before sleep increases so that sleep is less efficient.

These are questions a doctor will ask about a complaint of insomnia. How long has the condition been present? Are there symptoms of anxiety like heart palpitations, or other stress-related or depression symptoms? Does it feel like restless leg syndrome? Does he snore loudly or awaken at night gasping for air? Does he work a swing shift, or is he awakened by other stimuli during sleep? Is he rested when he awakens? Does he use prescription or non-prescription medicine or drugs? Does he use alcohol, caffeine in any form, or smoke?

Sleep Disorders
Sleep onset insomnia (not falling asleep)

Sleep maintenance insomnia (awakening after several hours and not going back to sleep)

Sleep apnea

Sleep Disorders (Continued)

Periodic limb movement

Restless leg syndrome

Disordered REM sleep

Narcolepsy

Night terrors

Idiopathic insomnia

Psychophysiologic insomnia

Jetlag

Sleep Apnea

Sleep apnea means loss of oxygen flow during sleep when the upper airway becomes partially obstructed from excess fat in the neck. Sleep disordered breathing may happen in 20% of men and is severe in 4% of them. During the night, the patient may rouse every few minutes just to get enough oxygen, resulting in severe sleep disruption. The sufferer then feels tired and tends to fall asleep during the day. Over time, severe sleep apnea can cause high blood pressure and heart disease including heart failure and heart rhythm abnormalities. Low testosterone levels, decreased libido and mental sluggishness may result from sleep apnea. Conversely, sleep apnea may be caused by an under active thyroid, rapid weight gain, testosterone supplements, and heart failure.

Sleep apnea is usually brought to the doctor's attention when a patient, or his spouse, describes these nighttime difficulties. The physical examination suggests sleep apnea if the person is overweight, has a receding chin, a deviated nasal septum, an elongated uvula and soft palate, excess tissue in the back of the throat, and large tonsils or tongue.

The diagnosis of sleep apnea is confirmed by observing the patient in a sleep laboratory. An audio monitor records snoring and the sound of obstructed breathing. Nasal and oral air flow measurements determine the presence of significant apnea (meaning cessation of air flow for ten seconds or more). Thoracic and abdominal muscular respiratory movements are monitored. If the person makes an effort to breathe with the diaphragm and there is no airflow within ten seconds, his or her airway is obstructed. If this happens more than 15 to 20 times an hour, it is significant. The severity of the problem is further defined by how long the apnea (lack of breathing) lasts and how low the blood oxygen dips. Pulse oximetry documents when the blood oxygen falls, and EEG (brain wave monitoring) tells us when the patient arouses from sleep and which stage of sleep he is in.

Weight loss improves sleep apnea by whittling away the excess layers of fat in the neck. A person may teach himself to lie on his side instead of his back and that may be as effective as more complex devices. Sleep apnea is only made worse with sedatives and alcohol just before going to bed. Some dental devices can maximize the airway. Nasal spray that decongests the nose or correction of a nasal septal deviation may bring relief. Sometimes the ENT surgeon can correct narrowed passages in the throat but these operations are only helpful in 50% of sleep apnea patients. Other times the patient must wear an apparatus called a CPAP (continuous positive airway pressure) machine with a facemask that keeps air flowing to the lungs throughout the night. The CPAP is not too popular with my patients, even when they really need it and at least half admit to discontinuing it. There are different types of masks (nasal mask, full-face, and other styles), and one may be more acceptable than another. Somehow, the romance of sleeping with someone seems diminished if one partner wears a noisy mask apparatus. Nonetheless, many people are able to resume sleeping in the same bed with their spouse despite the CPAP machine because the white noise generated by the equipment is more soothing than the snoring was.

Narcolepsy

Narcolepsy is a strange and poorly understood problem, with an estimated prevalence of 4 to 10 cases per 10,000 people in the United States. Symptoms usually start in the 20's and 30's and increase in severity through the third and fourth decade. The diagnosis is often delayed for years. Many doctors, when they hear the complaint of excessive daytime sleepiness, believe the patient is simply not getting enough sleep, but in true narcolepsy, that is not the problem. Classically, narcolepsy is an irresistible urge to sleep during daytime. These patients tend not to get more or less sleep than others, but they are unable to control passage from wakefulness to sleep and back again. Other symptoms include sleep paralysis, in which a person, upon awakening, may be unable to move for a few seconds or minutes, until touched by someone else, and cataplexy, a condition in which strong emotion such as anger, surprise, excitement or laughter suddenly weakens the muscles and, in some extreme cases, may cause a person to fall down. Cataplexy may also last a few seconds or several minutes. When brain wave recordings are done during cataplexy, we see a REM pattern in which all muscle action is inhibited, inserted into a waking moment. Frightening dreams when the patient is first transitioning into sleep are another symptom of this sleep disorder.

Narcolepsy is thought to be a problem of REM sleep. The first REM sleep normally starts about ninety minutes after onset of sleep, but in patients with narcolepsy, REM sleep begins within a few minutes.

The cause of narcolepsy may be a deficiency of hypocretin, a chemical in the brain that communicates the message to stay awake to the deepest part of the brain. Narcolepsy may run in families, since certain genes are more common in patients with this illness. Also, shift work can make narcolepsy worse. Conversely, regular sleeping and waking hours help patients.

Narcolepsy is treated with stimulant medicine. Ritalin, an amphetamine, was used for years, but the potential side effects of this drug are unpleasant, and include anxiety, palpitations, poor appetite and insomnia. A new medicine with the brand name of Provigil (chemical name modafinil) is now available. It is thought to work by raising the level of hypocretin in the brain. A person takes 200 to 400 mg. a day, and is usually able to stay awake without the side effects of an amphetamine, and with little addictive potential and no rise in blood pressure. Initially, Provigil may cause side effects such as headache or nausea, but these usually resolve after one week.

Periodic Limb Movement Disorder and Restless Leg Syndrome

Periodic limb movement disorder means clusters of repetitive toe, knee and hip motion during sleep. Some may be unaware of it and only experience daytime sleepiness. Restless leg syndrome happens at rest whether the person is asleep or not. Most that have restless leg syndrome also have the nighttime periodic limb movement disorder. Restless leg syndrome will develop in fifteen percent of us at some time in our lifetime, more commonly during middle and older age, and often as an inherited problem. Patients describe creeping sensations or compulsions to move the legs beginning shortly after going to bed. Movement and stretching temporarily relieve the symptoms, but they soon recur, often waking people. Restless leg syndrome may be associated with peripheral neuropathy (degeneration of the nerves of sensation of the legs), other neurologic problems, sleep apnea, and narcolepsy. The treatment is a benzodiazepam such as clonazepam, or Permax, Mirapex, or Requip, which enhance the chemical, dopamine, in the brain.

REM Sleep Behavior Disorder

This is an unusual but interesting problem in which the muscles are not paralyzed during dreams and the dreams get "acted out". The reported dream correlates closely with the action. (People may report fighting for their lives in dreams.) The muscles are supposed to be deeply relaxed during REM but are not in patients with this problem. These behaviors go far beyond the normal occasional twitching during sleep. Middle-aged and older males tend to have this condition as do those with other neurologic problems such as Parkinson's disease, stroke, or brain tumor. The newer anti-depressant medicines (SSRI's) may cause REM sleep behavior disorder in patients who never had it before. Pet animals have been observed with this problem. A videotape of the behavior during sleep shows how easily a person could hurt himself. The treatment is clonazepam. It works in 85% of cases, does not lose efficacy or require higher dosing with time, but the sleep disordered REM behavior recurs when clonazepam is stopped.

Other Sleep Disorders

Night terrors mean that a person gets a jolt of fight or flight symptoms, intense anxiety, heart palpitations, rapid breathing, and sweating in response to terrifying dreams. Alcohol and sleep deprivation make this worse. It is not due to an underlying psychiatric disorder like unexpressed anger. When observed in the sleep lab with an EEG (brain wave test), the terrors start very suddenly. Sometimes the person awakens or shifts to a lighter stage of sleep.

A genetic condition called familial fatal familial insomnia that affects ten to fifteen families begins with a complete inability to generate the brain waves of sleep and the victims die from it. This is probably closely related to Jacob Creutzfeldt disease in humans (mad cow disease in bovines.)

"Abduction by aliens" in seemingly normal people is a vivid

perception that usually happens halfway between sleep and waking. The victims usually are lying down, often trying to sleep when the aliens show up.

Difficulty Sleeping

People do not sleep as much as they did one hundred years ago. This trend accelerates as electricity, 24-hour days, and long commutes give people less time and more activities and demands. While the sleep disorders described above are fascinating, particularly narcolepsy with its associated cataplexy, my midlife patients often complain that they cannot fall asleep because their head is so full of things to do, unresolved issues and entropic events that they must right. The most common cause of poor sleep I see is daytime stress and worry. Sometimes people lie awake until two or three a.m., knowing that their full energy will be required the next day despite their sleepless state. When this happens, they become anxious and more awake. Sometimes they sedate themselves with alcohol, only to experience a rebound at 2 a.m. and an inability to go back to sleep. Depression also typically causes a person to awaken in the middle of the night or early in the morning and they are unable to go back to sleep. Traumatic events, such as the national tragedy on September 11, 2001, may disturb sleep in addition to causing fear, anxiety, and physical symptoms. Nightmares can make people afraid to go to sleep. Idiopathic insomnia is lifelong poor sleep. These people take longer to fall asleep, sleep less efficiently, and more frequently arouse with non-specific stimuli. They complain of daytime fatigue. Typically, people with insomnia have a faster pulse and more muscular tension than those who sleep more soundly, perhaps indicating that they are more influenced physically by the stresses of modern life.

Psychophysiologic insomnia is characterized by anxiety and focus on getting adequate sleep although the person can function the next day. These people tend to sleep better on vacation only to have a return of symptoms when the stressors are back. Self-relaxation, biofeedback, decreasing the amount of time in bed before attempting to sleep, hiding the clocks, leaving the bed when they are unable to sleep, or a low dose of a sedating anti-depressant may help.

Just as alcohol is an enemy of sound sleep, doctors also advise patients who have trouble sleeping to avoid all caffeine, including chocolate and caffeinated soft drinks. Cigarettes may act as a stimulant and should not be smoked within six hours of bedtime. Over-the-counter decongestants (such as sudafed or an antihistamine with a decongestant such as Claritin-D) can also act as a stimulant for many hours.

When a person exercises after 7 p.m., his body temperature may be too warm for falling asleep. He should exercise at least four hours before sleep to allow the body time to gradually cool off as bedtime approaches. Since sleep is associated with a cooling of the body, this may promote sounder sleep.

What Makes Insomnia Worse
Alcohol

Caffeine, including chocolate and soft drinks

Cigarettes within six hours of bedtime

Over-the-counter decongestants (containing D in name)

Drinking excessive fluids after dinner

A spouse's or pet's nocturnal habits

How to Sleep More Restfully
Go to bed only when you are ready to sleep.

Do not watch a clock in the bedroom.

Exercise before 7 p.m. to allow the body to cool.

Doctors tend not to prescribe sleeping medicines because patients get hooked on them. However, I have become more liberal in prescribing medicine such as clonazepam or Ambien (zolpidem) to normalize sleep patterns in patients who are sleeping poorly and are almost desperate about it. Sonata (zalepolon) lasts for four hours so a person can take it if wide awake at 2 a.m. and still be able to awaken refreshed in the morning. Although initially touted as non-addictive, Ambien and Sonata may cause dependency in some patients. I ask patients to use these medicines only when needed, not every night. Benadryl, an over-the-counter antihistamine, causes drowsiness. Two 25-mg. tablets will put most patients to sleep. This medication may also help their nighttime allergies. The side effects are a dry mouth and slowing of the urinary stream in men. Sometimes 50 mg. of benadryl can cause a hangover.

Other Medical Conditions That Contribute to Insomnia

Arthritis pains or bursitis may hurt more at night without the distractions of the day. Taking ibuprofen at bedtime (but not on an empty stomach) may help. Esophageal reflux or heartburn is classically worse during the night. An antacid at bedtime or Tagamet, Zantac Pepcid, or Prilosec may help. If the heartburn is so bad that over-the-counter preparations can't alleviate it, prescription medicine will help.

Nasal problems are a common cause of poor sleep. Nasal allergies may be worse during the night due to the airways' reaction to dust mites in the mattress and pillowcase. Dust mite coverings, and no carpet or pets in the bedroom are practical steps a sufferer might take. Steroid nasal inhalers such as Flonase or Nasacort AQ or Rhinocort often alleviate hay fever. Antihistamines such as benadryl or vistaril both ease allergic symptoms and put tired people to sleep. If the problem is a chronic infection of the sinuses causing a post-nasal drip and cough, it can be diagnosed by a CAT scan of the sinuses and treated with antibiotics. Nasal septal deviation gives patients the sensation of a blocked nostril and difficulty breathing through the upper airways, which gets worse at night. Otolaryngologists and plastic surgeons can straighten the septum. Polyps blocking the upper nasal passages can give a similar sensation of being unable to breathe through the nose at night. These too can be removed and recurrence prevented with nasal steroid inhalers. Patients addicted to Afrin or other nasal decongestants have a complicated problem and sleep poorly due to rebound nasal congestion.

Some patients complain about awakening at night to urinate and then being unable to fall back asleep. The technical term for this is nocturia. Nocturia may signal the onset of diabetes but more commonly, it is due to the prostate and urologic problems that normally appear in midlife. Nocturia is aggravated by drinking a lot of fluids with dinner and as the evening wears on. These are the practical tips I give my patients. They should avoid caffeine, which is a bladder stimulant. They should not drink excessive liquids after dinner. If possible, they should elevate their legs above the heart for an hour or two before going to sleep while they are watching television or reading. All people get a build-up of fluid in their legs during the day. If the fluid is pumped out via the heart and kidneys when they are trying to fall asleep, that can limit their hours of sound sleep. Leg elevation starts this diuresis process earlier in the evening.

Hormones and sleep are intricately related as the level of hormones varies throughout the day and night. This is the normal diurnal rhythm in all living things. People with thyroid and other hormonal disease tend to get insomnia.

Other Conditions That Cause Insomnia
Depression
Nasal obstruction from polyps or nasal septal deviation
Allergies from dust mites in pillows and mattresses

Other Conditions That Cause Insomnia (Continued)

Gastroesophageal reflux

Nocturia

Arthritis

A Sleep Issue We Do Not Talk About

Should couples always sleep in the same bedroom? Most are hesitant to even broach the subject because of the implications for loss of physical and emotional intimacy. However, sleep disturbances may be due to differences in sleep patterns between partners. One person may require eight hours of sleep while the other needs only six. One partner may work shifts and come to bed at various times, awakening the other. One partner may snore, thrash in the bed and talk in his or her sleep while the other may be sensitive to any disturbance and rouse easily from sleep. The result is that the lighter sleeper may often become sleep deprived. It is no myth that sleep deprivation makes people irritable. If a couple has the courage to openly discuss the subject, they may find they need to draw a distinction between sleep and sexual relations, and perhaps decide on separate bedrooms for sleeping.

A beloved cat or dog may disrupt sleep. Among pet owners who welcome their pet in the bedroom, over 50% are awakened nightly by them. These little darlings comfort us by being at our side during the night, but they make noise, and wake up to reassure themselves we are still there and doting on them. My cat, Amelia Earhart, requests a 4 a.m. snack from which she will not be deterred. Many people are willing to sacrifice sound sleep for the nighttime closeness of their pets.

Jetlag

I remember the first time I experienced jetlag. Mike and I went to India in 1985. At JKF airport in New York, we walked onto Air India. Beautiful air attendants with waist-length black hair, dressed in brilliantly colored saris with a third eye mark in the middle of their foreheads, pressed their palms together and said, "Namaste" to us. They were greeting our souls. We flew halfway around the world in twenty-four hours with very little sleep on a completely full jet. We arrived at the home of our gracious host on another short mid-morning flight after sitting through a night at the Bombay airport. The sisters of the family had me dress in a gauzy sari and took me directly to a bride shop to look at the most gorgeous 22-carat gold necklaces I had ever seen. That afternoon we listened to a sitar player as a gentle breeze passed through their upper porch. At bedtime, I was certain of falling deeply asleep and waking rested, but it was not to be. By midnight I was wide-awake, and stimulated by the Hindu culture, more fascinating than I had ever imagined.

Melatonin treats jetlag. It is a nutritional supplement that helps the body to adjust its natural rhythms to day and night. No amount of melatonin could have lessened my experience in India, but I have learned how to deal with jetlag in a more worldly way. For those flying east, take .5 mg melatonin at 2 p.m. the day before the trip. The day of an international flight, the traveler should board the plane, eat the dinner, and then tune out the airplane movie. He should put on a soft eye cover, blow up a neck pillow, and take 3-mg. of melatonin and a quick-acting sleeping tablet like Ambien (zolpidem) 10 mg. or Sonata (zalepolon) 10 mg. When the plane lands, exposure to sunlight tells the body that it is not 3 a.m. but rather morning. The traveler should stay up the rest of that day, and then go to bed at the usual time, according to the clock at the destination. Flying west, it may help to take .5 mg of melatonin in the morning the day before and the day of the flight. Late afternoon sunlight tells the brain it is not yet bedtime.

One word of caution about melatonin: They used to make it in Europe by extracting it from "bovine pineal glands." That means from the brains of the same cows that were dropping over from "mad cow disease." Many people no longer eat beef in Europe and you should check whether the melatonin is made from synthetic or "pharmacy grade" melatonin. Jetlag is one thing, but going to the grave with bovine spongiform encephalitis is another. Provigil, the newest drug for jetlag, helps the patient to be alert during the day. 200 mg. of Provigil in the morning cuts through some of the tiredness that normally affects people crossing two or more time zones.

Sound sleep is a great blessing. In Shakespeare's words:

"Sleep that knits up the raveled sleeve of care,
The death of each day's life, sore labor's bath,
Balm of hurt minds, great nature's second course,
Chief nourisher in life's feast."

How to Get Your Husband
in for a Check-up

When I talk about this book and solicit feedback from women I hear the same question. "How do I get my husband to go in for a check-up? He doesn't want to go to a doctor." Women usually go in for an annual Pap smear and renewal of their oral contraceptive prescription, but a man may not have seen the doctor since childhood when he broke his leg or received immunizations.

Men in our society are trained to be stoic through participation in sports and later in military service. It is part of manly culture not to admit physical weakness. The notion of going to the doctor is likely to meet with resistance at first. Nowhere is this more flagrant than among military pilots, where going to the doctor is synonymous with getting grounded. When I was in the Air Force, a tough, fearless general officer patient called me from a base in Korea before I saw him for the first time. He wanted me to know he had no problems but would see me since his wife needed a physical examination and he was willing to accompany her back to the U.S.

My own husband, Mike, had skin cancers on his face in his late thirties because of his pink Irish complexion. After asking him several times to see the dermatologist, I finally told the retired officer who ran his clinic that Mike needed time off for his "cancer treatment" and I made the appointment. This was hardball, but it worked. The wife often recognizes that her husband has not seen his doctor in a long time and that he is overestimating how healthy he really is. It is my hope that this book will help a man and his wife get a handle on the specific issues he and his doctor are likely to go over and make the problem of going to the doctor seem smaller.

One strategy is to appeal to his sense of duty and responsibility; his family loves him and needs him to stay around, so he should visit his doctor to stay healthy. If he even hints that he might like to get a check-up sometime, or that his father had a heart attack five years later than his current age, it means you should make the appointment. If he counters that it may be an expense, remind him that he is covered by the company health plan.

Men are more likely to desire an overhaul when a friend or relative has a heart attack or cancer. Many of my patients feel motivated to improve themselves after the beginning of the New Year and that would be another opportunity to get him in for a check-up. The wife could spin it a little, as in "Would you rather go to a man or a lady doctor?" Or, "Do you want to see my internal medicine doctor or should I make the appointment with another doctor in our health plan?" Going in for a check-up may be equated with getting a tune-up for his car, something he will do without a second thought. Sports metaphors such as problem solving, teamwork, and goal setting, are words that make men feel in control of a situation.

If you do get your husband to agree to see his doctor, be sure you have scheduled thirty minutes so that the doctor can address all relevant issues in that one visit. Four p.m. is not the best time because the doctor is more likely to be running over time with another patient's urgent problem by then. Often, that visit will be the first interaction with a health care professional a man will have had in over ten years.

Men Hate Side Effects

I have described medicines that make men live longer and better lives. So why don't they take them? Because they are afraid they will have side effects. The most feared side effect is a detrimental effect on sexual function. But there are others that you need to know about in case he does end up on a few of these medicines and starts complaining about something new.

The medicines that may cause sexual side effects are all anti-depressants except for Wellbutrin (buproprion), and the classes of blood pressure medicine including diuretics, beta blockers, and centrally acting drugs (almost always used in older adults and not middle-aged people.) Sometimes Propecia, a medicine used for male pattern balding, blocks testosterone. Rarely, Tagamet does that. In contrast, ACE inhibitors and ARB type drugs for high blood pressure dilate the blood vessels and the statins for cholesterol clean out the blood vessels and promote the rapid inflow of blood, both of which may help erectile function.

I would be cautious about calling the doctor and asking for an antibiotic prescription every time your husband gets a cold. Most colds are viral and do not respond to antibiotics. I stopped prescribing antibiotics with sulfa because the allergic reactions can be too severe. I do not prescribe Augmentin, a potent penicillin, for sinusitis, because it causes so many gastrointestinal side effects, although my colleagues still use it as an effective antibiotic for bad infections. One of the worst gastrointestinal side effects to antibiotics, particularly amoxicillin or cephalosporin, is clostridia difficile diarrhea. Clostridia difficile is a diarrhea/colitis causing bacteria that is allowed to grow in the intestine when the good bacteria are wiped out by an antibiotic directed at another part of the body. It has spores, so just when you think you have it cleared up, the spores may hatch, and it comes back, over and over, for up to a year.

Cholesterol medicine may cause muscle aching, but this is diffuse, not just a sore shoulder or back. Anti-inflammatories used for arthritis and aches and pains may cause gastritis and bleeding ulcers in the worst case. They may also cause canker sores in his mouth. The stomach side effects of arthritis medicine can be ameliorated by taking the medicine with meals. The arthritis pills also can raise blood pressure and cause feet swelling. Anti-histamines like benadryl or the old anti-depressants like nortriptylline can cause the sphincter at the outlet of his bladder to go into spasm and he may not be able to urinate well or at all.

Headaches can be a side-effect of almost any medicine. Over the years, I have watched my husband get disabling headaches from arthritis medicine and some of the newer, stronger ACE inhibitors for blood pressure. He still takes an ACE inhibitor, captopril, the first one on the market in the mid 80's and tolerates it well. I have had severe headaches from Zantac and Pepcid. So if he starts something new, then mentions his new headaches, think about a possible side effect.

Charlie Makes an
Appointment to See Me

We return to Charlie from the first chapter. Charlie is in my office at 8 a.m. I ask him what brings him in today. He says he doesn't know, that his wife made him come in for a physical. I ask him if he has any problems. He says, "No." We talk about his past medical and surgical history, then his family history. I notice that his father died young of a heart attack. I ask Charlie if he has ever had chest pain, discomfort, burning, or a funny feeling in his jaws or shoulders when he exerts himself. He says, "No." I do a complete physical examination including a prostate and rectal exam. I check his cholesterol, triglycerides, HDL, LDL (a complete lipid profile), lipoprotein (a), homocysteine, and highly sensitive C-reactive protein level because his father had premature coronary artery disease. I check a fasting blood sugar to screen for diabetes. For cancer screening, he gets a PSA, a blood test for prostate cancer and is scheduled for a colonoscopy (under intravenous sedation).

When the tests come back, his total cholesterol is elevated at 240 mg/dl (less than 200 is normal), and his HDL, or protective type of cholesterol, is low at 30mg/dl (it should be over 35). His lipoprotein (a) level is 84 (normal should not be above 30). I think he needs a stress test and luckily, they are able to do it that afternoon.

I can see Charlie getting more and more leery that he is going down this medical slippery slope. He wishes he had not even started. He has enough to worry about. Still, I must keep him engaged in what we are doing. I have a bad feeling based on his family history and lipids that he has premature coronary disease. Sure enough, the stress test is positive. We sit and talk that over and I spend as much time as it takes to listen and answer questions. I call the chairman of cardiology who says he would be happy to talk with him. I tell Charlie without equivocating that it is possible that he has coronary disease, that a catheterization will tell us if he needs to have a blood vessel opened with a stent, and that whatever the findings at catheterization, we need to aggressively manage his cholesterol problem.

He has the catheterization and because of the sedation, it isn't so bad and he doesn't really remember the procedure. He does have a significant blockage in one coronary artery and the cardiologist stents it open. Charlie returns to me to manage his cholesterol and other factors contributing to premature atherosclerotic plaque.

By now Charlie is taking it pretty well, and he no longer denies having anything that could possibly merit medical attention. He tells me, after the fact, that he had 30 minutes of chest pain two weeks ago, took Maalox without relief, then forgot about it. To treat his cholesterol, I prescribe Pravachol 40 mg. at bedtime. He also needs to take Ecotrin 81 mg. daily, (a coated baby aspirin), a one gram capsule of fish oil and Folgard or Foltx (folic acid and vitamin B combination daily.) I schedule a follow-up visit in one month at which time we will repeat his lipid profile and check his liver and muscle function. We also need to plan a healthier diet, weight loss, and an aerobic exercise program, now that it is safe for him to start exercising without risk of a heart attack.

I will see Charlie periodically for the next six months and in time we will get to the issue of two Scotches a night, the life troubles in the last two years, his insomnia, and whether a prescription for Viagra may be helpful. His blood pressure is borderline, so after seeing how he does with weight loss, we will decide if he needs an ACE inhibitor to lower his blood pressure; he probably does.

So now we are at the end. I have covered the most common physical and emotional problems that happen to our husbands at midlife. It is surprising how you can feel age 20 one day and realize you are really 50 the next. I hope this book has made the whole experience of a man going to the doctor seem less threatening and more within the normal bounds of living.

GLOSSARY

Cardiology terms:

Atherosclerosis means cholesterol laden plaque that may narrow blood vessels.

Coronary artery disease means atherosclerotic plaque in the vessels of the heart.

HDL is the "good kind" of cholesterol carrier; it removes plaque from arteries.

LDL is the "bad kind" of cholesterol carrier; it delivers cholesterol to the walls of the arteries.

Highly sensitive C-reactive protein is a measure of inflammation in blood vessels.

Inflammation means activation of a person's own immune cells.

Homocysteine is a part of a protein that contributes to atherosclerosis and stroke.

Lipoprotein (a) is a bad kind of inherited cholesterol that works with high LDL to cause heart attacks.

Triglycerides are another blood fat that can cause atherosclerosis.

An **unstable atherosclerotic plaque** is bloated with cholesterol and prone to rupture.

A **stable atherosclerotic plaque** may not do anything.

A **thrombus** is a clump of platelets that block the blood vessel suddenly at the site of a ruptured atherosclerotic plaque.

Hypertension is the same thing as high blood pressure.

Atrial fibrillation is an irregular heart rhythm that can cause blood clots that cause stroke.

A **heart catheterization** is the same as an angiogram; dye is put in to the coronary arteries.

A **stress EKG** is an electrical tracing while the heart is pumping harder with exercise.

A **stress echo** is both an electrical tracing and an image of the heart by ultrasound while it is pumping harder with exercise.

A **stress nuclear scan** is another way to image the heart with exercise.

A **stent** is used to prop open a closing coronary artery after it is dilated.

Coronary artery disease means atherosclerotic plaque in the vessels of the heart.

Weight and diet problems:

BMI is the percent of body fat; an alternate to measuring pounds for weight control.

Monounsaturated fats like olive oil are best for blood vessels.

Saturated fat that is solid at room temperature can add to cholesterol plaque.

Sleep problems:

Sleep apnea is when the upper airway blocks off during sleep.

Restless leg syndrome is a crawling feeling in the legs asleep or awake. It is called periodic limb movement when people are asleep.

Disordered REM sleep is when people act out their dreams.

Urology terms:

Benign prostatic hypertrophy is enlargement that all men get with age, of the prostate gland at the base of the bladder.

Prostatitis is infection or inflammation of the prostate gland.

Books by Whiskey Hollow Press:

The Other Midlife Crisis:
Arthritis and All Those Aches and Pains
By Michael R. Wilson, M.D., Orthopedic Surgeon

Dispatches From the Frontlines of Medicine:
Your Husband's Health:
Simplify Your Worry List
By Kathleen Wilson, M.D.

Coming Soon...

Dispatches From the Frontlines of Medicine:
By Kathleen Wilson, M.D.

For Women:
When You Feel Like You Are Falling Apart

Maintain Your Brain!
Preventing Stroke and Dementia

When One Thing Leads to Another:
Critical Turning Points in the Health of Older Parents

Where is Marcus Welby When We Need Him?
Managing in the Medical System

Soul Survival:
Midlife Medicine for African Americans
By Giselle Wilson and Kathleen Wilson, M.D.

Midlife Medicine Series

Qty	Title	Price
	The Other Midlife Crisis: Arthritis and All Those Aches and Pains ISBN 0-9742976-0-7	$21.95
	Dispatches from the Frontlines of Medicine: Your Husband's Health: Simplify Your List ISBN 0-9742976-1-5	$14.95
	Subtotal	
	Sales Tax (if applicable)	
	Shipping and Handling ($4.00 U.S./$14.00 International)	
	TOTAL	

Shipping Address

Name _____

Address _____

City_____ State_____ Zip Code_____

Country_____

Telephone_____ Fax_____ E-mail_____

Billing Address (if different from shipping)

Name _____

Address _____

City_____ State_____ Zip Code_____

Country_____

Name as it appears on your credit card_____

Credit card#_____cid#_____

Order by fax, mail or online:

Whiskey Hollow Press
P.O. Box 13752 • New Orleans, LA 70185-3752
(504) 861-2188 • Fax (504) 861-1657
www.boomermedicine.com
www.whiskeyhollowpress.com

Shipping time is usually 3-5 business days.